PUFFIN BOOKS

The Other Facts of Life

Morris Gleitzman was born and educated in England. He went to Australia with his family in 1969 and studied for a degree. In 1974 he began work with the ABC, left to become a full-time film and television writer in 1978 and has written numerous television scripts. He has two children and lives in Sydney, but visits England regularly. One of the best-selling children's authors in Australia, his first children's book was *The Other Facts of Life*, based on his award-winning screenplay. This was followed by the highly-acclaimed *Two Weeks with the Queen* and *Bumface,* amongst others.

Other books by Morris Gleitzman,

BUMFACE
GIFT OF THE GAB
SECOND CHILDHOOD
TOTALLY WICKED!
TWO WEEKS WITH THE QUEEN

Morris Gleitzman

The Other Facts of Life

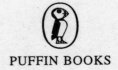

PUFFIN BOOKS

PUFFIN BOOKS

Published by the Penguin Group
Penguin Books Ltd, 27 Wrights Lane, London W8 5TZ, England
Penguin Putnam Inc., 375 Hudson Street, New York, New York 10014, USA
Penguin Books Australia Ltd, Ringwood, Victoria, Australia
Penguin Books Canada Ltd, 10 Alcorn Avenue, Toronto, Ontario, Canada M4V 3B2
Penguin Books (NZ) Ltd, Private Bag 102902, NSMC, Auckland, New Zealand

On the World WideWeb at: www.penguin.com

Penguin Books Ltd, Registered Offices: Harmondsworth, Middlesex, England

First published by McPhee Gribble Publishers Australia 1985
Published in Australia in Puffin Books 1993
7 9 10 8

Made and printed in England by Clays Ltd, St Ives plc

British Library Cataloguing in Publication Data
A CIP catalogue record for this book is available from the British Library

ISBN 0–140–36877–9

For Sophie and the other Ben

1

GRASPING THE GRISTLE

It was a beautiful Saturday morning but inside the bathroom things weren't so good.

Ben stared at himself in the mirror. The Feeling was coming on again. It was coming every day now, sometimes more than once a day. And it was getting stronger.

It was already stronger than the feeling he got unwrapping presents. Stronger than the dentist's waiting room feeling. Even stronger than those mornings he fell out of bed feeling twenty-three instead of twelve and Mum hit him with sausages for breakfast.

Ben had never felt a feeling like this in his life.

He needed answers. He stared into the mirror at the plump, pink flesh sitting all over his body. It had been with him for a while and he thought he knew it pretty well. Bruised from footy. Scraped from bike falls. Freckled from eating curry.

But now it was asking him questions he'd never heard before. And he needed answers.

Quickly.

Outside the bathroom Ben's mother wanted answers too. Pressing her ear to the door, she held her breath. What was he doing in there?

Di Guthrie had a quick vision of what she herself was doing and felt guilty. Sneaking around the house listening at doors wasn't the way they usually did things in this family. But Ben had been shutting himself in there at least once a day for the last two weeks. Sometimes twice. On top of the normal wees, poos and showers.

One thing was certain. He wasn't retiling the floor. Not after what she'd just found in his room.

Outside the house, the bush suburb was auditioning for a margarine commercial. Sunlight filtered through the tall gums, bathing the big new houses in golden light. Swimming pools glowed through brushwood fencing. Lawns sparkled under their whispering sprinklers.

On every side Substantial Pieces of Real Estate sat around increasing in value. Nobody was getting mugged, all the drugs were safely stored in generously proportioned bathroom cabinets, the only hints of unemployment were a couple of discreet For Sale signs.

In Crescents, Closes and Places, remote-controlled triple garage doors whirred open. Golden haired kids zipped up their leather moto-cross suits, kick-started their shiny Yamahas and Kawasakis and roared away into the bush in clouds of blue smoke and happy laughter.

But not Ben.

Why me? he thought as he stared into the mirror. Why not the other kids? Or has it happened to them and they just haven't noticed?

I've always been pretty observant, thought Ben. I get it from Dad. He's always been pretty observant.

Dad stood on the driveway in front of the house of his dreams not seeing a brick of it.

He spread waves of soapy water from the Swirl-On over his late model airconditioned Fairlane without seeing that either.

Nor was he seeing the Mazda hatchback, the eight metre cabin cruiser on its trailer, the four surf skis or the four trail bikes all lined up across the driveway, all as yet untouched by soapy water.

What he was seeing was meat. Lamb, beef and pork. Dressed, chilled and hanging in rows that stretched away as far as his inner eye could see.

This wasn't as much of a problem as it could have been because Ron Guthrie was a butcher. And the voice coming from the car radio was reading out the most important items of information in Ron's day. The abattoir prices.

'. . . young cattle dressed weight medium number three a hundred and ninety-eight cents to two hundred and four cents average two hundred and one cents . . .'

Ron Swirled On, his work-weary face furrowed with concentration, oblivious to the soapy water that splashed onto his footy shirt and shorts, onto his paunch and his pale legs.

On neighbouring driveways other tired, overweight men in ironed football gear soaped down their own lineups of cars, boats, bikes and other luxury hardware. Those that weren't gliding hover-mowers over already manicured lawns. Or running power clippers over immaculate hedges.

Several of them looked over as Ben's mother hurried out of the Guthrie house and down the driveway to her husband. Trim and tanned in her tennis dress, her pretty, well-cared-for face furrowed, Di didn't give them a glance. All she cared about was the thing she held in her hand.

A magazine. Glossy. With a naked woman on the front. Well, almost naked. The magazine, *National Geographic*, showed on its cover a statuesque African tribeswoman bare from the waist up, her breasts half-obscured by strands

4

of tribal jewellery.

Di held the magazine out to Ron. He glanced at it distractedly, ears still tuned to the radio, mind still juggling carcasses and prices per kilo.

'Mmm . . . very nice,' he murmured absently. 'Necklace'll go with your Mexican earrings.'

Di thrust the magazine under his nose. She tried to sound calm.

'I found it in Ben's room.'

At that moment the voice on the radio announced a dramatic fall in the price of pork. Ron winced the wince of a man with a freezer full of porcine stiffs bought at last week's record prices.

Di decided to ignore the soapy water filling Ron's sandshoes and continue.

'He's in there again now. When a twelve-year-old boy starts shutting himself away on sunny Saturday mornings with videotapes and photos of naked women it can only mean one thing.'

Ron, in the process of weighing a special on pork sausages against a pork chop promotion, became dimly aware that Di was waiting for him to say something.

'Ummm . . . what's that?' he said.

Di felt a surge of irritation as she realized the most important moment in her son's life was coming second to a bunch of dead pigs. She leant forward and whispered fiercely.

'Sex.'

Ron, crouching closer to the radio – things

5

weren't looking much better in the grain-fed beef department – became aware he'd just missed an important word.

'Eh?' he ventured.

Di could hold it in no longer.

'SEX!'

Her shout echoed down the street.

Ron snapped upright, soapy water arching through the sunlight and pattering onto his thinning scalp.

The washers, mowers and clippers for several houses around looked up in alarm. Seeing their footy shorts were not under immediate threat they bent back down to their tasks for fear of becoming involved in a Domestic.

Ron grabbed the magazine, stared at the cover and put Ben, the semi-naked tribeswoman and Di's concern together in a flash. His stomach gave a little lurch.

Leaning past him into the car, Di turned off the radio and looked at him.

'It's time you had a chat with him, Ron,' she said quietly.

Ron felt a sudden urge to go to each of his four butcher's shops and proclaim the special on pork sausages in person. He glanced at his watch.

'I will,' he said. 'I will. Soon.'

'Now. He's twelve. Jean and Barry did the birds and the bushflies with Jason months ago.'

'You're right, love. It's just I'm a bit flat out this morning. Don't s'pose you . . .?'

Di put her hands on his shoulders and sharply lifted her knee to within one centimetre of his groin.

'I did Claire, you do Ben. That was the deal.' She stepped back, exasperated. 'I mend his football. I tune his bike. I teach him karate. He's been waiting years for this just so he can get to see you.'

Ron swirled the soapy water around on the car roof, feeling guilty and resentful at the same time.

'I've got a business to run. If I spent all my time tuning his bike we wouldn't be able to afford to buy him one. Besides, the bottom's fallen out of pigs.'

Di took the Swirl-On from him. 'The shops can wait for once.' She pointed to the row of vehicles. 'I'll finish these.'

Ron felt the old panic surge through him. Never enough time. Supermarkets discounting behind his back, leaving him with windows full of stock fit only for currying. Mortgages collapsing around him. Family leaving him, bowels ravaged by tonnes of Vindaloo. He looked gloomily at his drivewayful of possessions.

'What's the use of owning all this stuff if I haven't got time to clean it?'

Di slipped her arm round his waist and gave him a sympathetic squeeze.

'Go on, Ron. Go in and sort it all out with him so he can get back out on his bike with his mates.'

On cue Ben's mates roared past on their bikes, leaving behind them a trail of smoke, laughter and credit repayments.

Ron looked at his watch. 'Have to be a quick chat.'

He started moving uncertainly towards the house. Di watched him go.

'Couple of minutes should be plenty,' she called after him with gentle sarcasm. 'It's only the Facts of Life.'

In the darkness of his bedroom, curtains shutting out the sunlight, Ben sat huddled in front of his TV.

A cassette turned slowly in his video player.

The frenzied, pulsating beat of oriental drums filled the room.

Ben stared at the images on the screen half in fascination, half in horror.

He had never seen anything like this.

It was incredible.

It was awful.

He needed answers.

2

CHEWING THE FAT

'. . . and in conclusion . . .'
    '. . . gurgle, gurgle . . .'
    '. . . if there's anything you'd like to ask . . .'
    '. . . gurgle, gurgle . . .'
    '. . . no matter how intimate or personal . . .'
Ron took a deep breath. This wasn't so bad.
The words were even coming out in the right
order. He tried to get a bit more wise, understanding fatherliness into his voice. Bit more
Obi Wan Kenobi.
    '. . . anything about yourself . . .'
    '. . . gurgle, gurgle . . .'
    '. . . or me . . .'
    '. . . gurgle, gurgle . . .'
    '. . . or your sister . . .'
    '. . . gurgle, gurgle . . .'
    '. . . or your mother . . .'
    '. . . gurgle, gurgle . . .'
    '. . . don't hesitate, don't hold back, don't
beat around the bush . . .'
    The automatic pool cleaner didn't beat around
the bush. It just carried on crawling around the
pool, sucking up dead leaves and insects with a
rhythmic gurgle, blissfully untroubled by

intimate or personal questions about its immediate family.

Ron stopped his pacing around the pool. Di was looking at him from the kitchen window. He gave her a little wave and hurried into the house.

Not a bad rehearsal. Now for the real thing.

Ben knew his life was changed forever almost thirty seconds before he heard the knock on his door. Sitting cross-legged on his floor in the gloom, staring unblinking at the people moving on the TV screen, he felt the Feeling growing in him stronger than ever and knew things would never be the same.

Knock, knock on the door. Ben decided whoever it was he was going to try for some answers. He hit the remote control and the screen went blank. The door opened slightly and Ron, wearing a safari business suit, peered in.

'G'day. Can I come in?'

He came in.

Ben got to his feet and started to open the curtains. Sunlight spilled in onto the bright, modern furniture.

'Don't get up,' said Ron.

Don't get up? Ben had only ever heard Dad say this to pensioners. He knew there were no pensioners in the room. He sat back down on the floor and pushed his glasses up his nose.

Ron sat down next to him, lowering his backside as if half expecting the Berber carpet to bite him. He tried to cross his legs. The shorts of his safari business suit creaked in protest. Ron thought better of it and sat uncomfortably with his legs apart, his elbows on his knees.

'How are things?' he said.

'Fine,' said Ben, because all the things he desperately wanted to say had scrambled in his head. He hoped they sewed safari suits with nylon thread. 'How are things with you?'

'You know the meat business,' said Ron. 'Bloody murder.'

Ben laughed. This was one of Dad's Jokes and Ben always did the right thing and laughed. Except today it didn't come out right so he changed it to a cough. He wondered what was going on.

Ron shifted from one buttock to the other and stared into the distance. Or would have done if there hadn't been a wall covered with framed moto-cross action posters in the way.

'Talking of the meat business,' he said casually, his voice giving the tiniest little quaver. 'You know son, when a butcher's chopping up an animal it's not all rump and topside. There are bits of an animal we don't talk about very much . . .'

'Like kidneys?' All Ben wanted to do at this moment was put his father at his ease. He wished they were sitting on chairs. Or wearing looser clothes.

11

Ron's face fell. 'Yeah . . . kidneys.' This wasn't the response from Ben he'd rehearsed by the pool. He pressed on.

'Um . . . look Ben old mate, you've reached an age now where there are probably some pretty tricky questions bothering you and . . . well, I'm going to answer them for you now. Anything at all. Anything that, just for example, may have to do with any tapes you may have seen lately, say.'

Ben's heart kicked him in the chest. The Busiest Man In The World had actually come to him, in his room, and had just asked him the one thing in the world he most desperately wanted to be asked. If he hadn't been scared of knocking him over he would have hugged his Dad.

'Is there anything?'

'Yes,' said Ben, 'there is.'

Ron wriggled his blood-starved buttocks and spoke with all the bravado of a condemned man without a blindfold staring down a row of rifle barrels.

'Great, great. Fire away.'

Ben looked his father in the eyes. 'Why are so many people in the world starving?'

Ron stared blankly at his son.

'What?'

Ben tried to carve each word into marble with his mouth.

'How come so many people in the world are starving?'

Ron felt as though his head was full of fluttering birds and bees.

'Starving? What's that got to do with . . .?'

Ben hit the remote control, the video player clicked on and the TV screen glowed into life.

A dry, flat, sun-scorched plain. Hundreds of people in loose cotton clothes crouching in the dust. Some wearing only loincloths. Thin bodies. Gaunt faces. Hopeless eyes staring out of the screen.

Ron stared back, stunned. A reporter's voice broke through the frenzied Indian drums.

'. . . The famine has already claimed tens of thousands of lives. Hundreds of thousands more will not survive the summer. In the time it takes you to watch this film, dozens of babies will die.'

Men and women, their bodies shrivelled, huddled together in family groups. Their children just sitting, dull-faced, stomachs swollen, arms and legs like kite-struts. A mother holding a tiny, still baby.

Ron leant forward and touched the remote control. The screen went blank. Ron's body sagged.

'Is that what you've been looking at, stuck away in here?' he said gently. Ben nodded. Ron put his hand on his son's head and ruffled his hair.

'Mate,' he said, his voice soft with relief, 'you don't have to worry about all that. There are huge, well-organized charities taking care of all that.'

Ben struggled for words to express the Feeling that welled up inside him. Come on, dummo, now's your chance.

'But Dad . . .'

But Ron was already staggering to his feet, wincing as the blood rushed painfully into his numb buttocks.

'Vast, highly-trained organizations,' he said, half his mind already grappling with pork sausages.

He glanced at his watch and looked apologetically at Ben.

'I've obviously got the wrong end of the stick here. Your mum thinks you've got some hoard of magazines tucked away . . .'

He gave Ben a shrug. Saying they both knew what mothers were like. This is it, thought Ben, all or nothing. He got up, went to his cupboard and pulled out a pile of magazines. Ron's face dropped. Apart from his backside, which felt like it had been injected with Fanta, his body tensed.

And relaxed again when he saw that the magazines were all copies of *Time* and other news publications. He took them from Ben and flicked through the pile.

Every cover story was on war, famine, pollution or nuclear catastrophe. The Hidden War. Our Dying Planet. A Nation Mourns. Eve of Destruction.

Quite a collection, thought Ron. Whatever happened to stamps?

Once again he ruffled Ben's hair.

'Mate,' he said gently, 'these are American magazines. The whole nuclear thing's between America and Russia.'

Ben looked at him steadily. Come on, Dad, he thought, I'm not ten.

Ron straightened his back and spoke in the voice he'd planned to use if he ever found himself Prime Minister.

'Now look, you haven't really caught my drift here and it's probably my fault so I'm going to be blunt. Man to man. Is there anything you want to ask, as intimate or personal as you like, about yourself, or your sister, or . . . or me . . . or even your mother?'

Ben looked him straight in the eyes.

'Yes, Dad,' he said, 'there is.'

Ron took a deep breath, swallowed and licked his lips.

Ben pointed to the pile of magazines.

'How can we carry on living happily with all this going on?'

The air trickled out of Ron. His safari business suit seemed to be two sizes bigger.

'A . . . e . . . i . . .'

Ron tried to form an answer but the words wouldn't come. He looked at his watch and took on the appearance of a man with a serious sausage problem to solve.

'Look . . . er . . . perhaps you'd better ask your mum.'

Ben watched his father hurry out of the room.

Typical, he thought. I ask him a serious question and all he wants to talk about is sex.

Ben stood in front of the bathroom mirror stripped to the waist. He flexed his biceps and tried to wiggle his pectorals. The muscles sat snugly in their warm flesh coat.

Ben looked down at the magazine lying on the sink. Staring up at him from a page was a boy his own age. A refugee boy stripped to the waist like him.

Under his skin the refugee boy's skeleton appeared to be held together by rubber bands.

Ben looked back at his own pink flesh. He wished the whole thing wasn't happening. As well as everything else it was ruining his social life.

Okay, he'd been pretty stupid to bring it up at a Satan's Spaceriders Club meeting. He remembered the blank looks when he asked the others if they ever worried about people starving overseas. Then the sneering laughter that rang through the stormwater drain.

Then Angus Skinner had said he only worried about himself starving in Double Chemistry and the others laughed themselves sick. If Skinner wasn't only eleven Ben would have nutted him. Instead he tried to explain.

But they'd all blasted their bike horns at him which was the ultimate Spacerider insult.

16

Then they chucked him out of the club for being soft.

Ben looked at the boy in the magazine, at the sores on his face, at the folds of skin under his ribs, at the misshapen joints on his hands and hoped from his own tousled blond hair to the tips of his pink toes that Mum had some answers.

3

BEN'S BEEF

Claire Guthrie keeled over and crashed to the kitchen floor. She lay motionless, eyes closed, arms splayed.

Instead of sprinting to the phone, ringing an ambulance, sprinting back, giving Claire mouth-to-mouth, weeping, panicking and making silly deals with God, her mother merely sighed and plonked down a steak the size of Tasmania onto the kitchen table in front of Ben.

'Claire,' said Di, long-sufferingly.

Ben wasn't too worried by his sister's collapse either. He thought she'd held the horrified stare at her plate a couple of seconds too long and one roll of the eyes before going down would have done but at that moment he was more interested in beef than ham. He stared thoughtfully at the two huge steaks steaming on the table.

Claire's eyes snapped open and she dragged herself theatrically onto her chair.

'Sorry,' she said, 'it was just too much for me, the sight of three months' meals all on the one plate.'

'Eat your lunch,' said Di sharply.

Claire sat up and cleared her throat.

'Here is the news. A sixteen-year-old girl stuffed three months' meals into herself today and couldn't walk until a Japanese whaling ship cut the blubber off with bulldozers . . .'

Di thumped a bowl of potato salad down onto the table and struggled to control her anger.

'Claire . . .'

Claire's shoulders drooped and her eyes filled with tears. She stood up and looked down at her slim figure.

'You don't care that I'm fat,' she mumbled.

With a whoosh Di's steak burst into flames under the grill. Di grabbed a tea-towel and began swatting at it, calling to Claire over her shoulder.

'Lots of people in the world would give anything for that steak.'

A couple more swats and Di lifted her own smoking acreage of meat from her self-cleaning, self-fan-forcing but unfortunately not self-extinguishing cooker.

She turned to see Claire storming out of the kitchen and closed her eyes, wishing she'd handled things differently.

Ben looked up from his thoughtful scrutiny of the steaks. This was going to be lousy timing but he had to do it.

'Why do we have so much meat?' he asked.

Di became the second thing to flare up in the

19

kitchen that morning.

'Because,' she yelled, slamming her steak onto its plate, 'we own four butcher's shops and if a constant supply of the best steak isn't good enough for you then I'm terribly sorry, we'll try and make the next one caviar.'

Ben frowned helplessly, pushing his glasses up his nose.

'No, I mean why do we have so much meat when half the world's starving?'

Before Di could answer, Claire stormed back into the kitchen. She slapped a padded post bag onto the table, scrawled 'The Poor People' on the front of it with a marker pen, snatched the steak from her plate, dropped it into the bag, stapled the bag closed, dropped the bag onto the table and stormed out.

Di sank wearily into a chair.

'Ben, I can't think about the rest of the world, I've got enough to worry about here. A daughter who thinks she's a whale, a husband determined to work himself into a early grave, you stuck in your room with R-rated magazines, one of the airconditioners has blown up, two of the bikes are out of rego, the rotisserie in the microwave won't go round . . .'

Ben cut in animatedly.

'But you just said to Claire that lots of people in the world would give anything for her steak. That's thinking about the rest of the world.'

'It's a figure of speech,' said Di softly. 'It's what mothers say instead of "eat that steak you ungrateful little shit or I'll stuff it down your throat with a curling wand".'

Ben went over to the work surface and picked up the *National Geographic*. He opened it at an article on drought in Ethiopia and held the pages in front of his mother.

'Mum, how can we ignore this?' he asked. There, the Big One. But Mum could handle it. God, death, pimples. She'd never shied away from a big question in the past.

Di looked at the emaciated children staring uncomprehendingly out from the pages.

'Is this what you got this for?' she said in amazement. She turned back to the bare-breasted tribeswoman on the cover. 'Not this?'

'No,' said Ben, puzzled. 'That's a different article. Water conservation in West Africa.'

He took back the magazine and turned back to the Ethiopia pages.

'The drought's in Ethiopia. East Africa.' God, she could be thick for someone who did a year of uni. Well, nine months.

Di took back the magazine and turned back to the cover.

'You don't find this more interesting?' she said, with growing concern.

'No,' said Ben. What was this fixation with water conservation? A hint about him leaving the shower running?

Di held the cover slightly closer to him.

'There's nothing special that strikes you about this woman . . . physically?'

21

The tribeswoman's teak brown breasts heaved with his mother's anxiety.

Double homework, he thought, her as well. Give a bloke a break – my voice hasn't even broken yet. So that's what all the fuss with sex was about. He'd known it was for more than just having babies. Now all had been revealed. The reason adults were obsessed with sex was that it stopped them having to think about the suffering, misery and impending disaster that screamed at them from every side.

Ben realized his mother was waiting for him to respond to the tribeswoman's physical bits.

'She's better fed. They probably get more rain in West Africa.'

He looked at Di sadly.

Di smiled weakly, suddenly concerned that Ben shouldn't realize he was a late developer and get neurotic about it. She made a mental note to give him more meat.

Claire shivered with anticipation as the warm Hollywood breeze caressed her skin. She allowed herself a slow, smouldering glance across the blinding strip of Sunset Boulevard to where the figures stood nonchalantly around the black sports car. Five tanned young men, each one the star of a major motion picture.

'Oh poop bum!'

Okay, it wasn't actually Hollywood, but

when you're stuck in a Sydney bush suburb miles from the city you do what you can with five shops and a service station.

Claire allowed herself another slow, smouldering glance across the blinding strip of Wattle Parade to the five tanned young men standing around Des Turkle's mother's black hatchback.

'Poop poop poop.'

Her friend Amanda hissed furiously as she slipped a long, laquered nail under a small piece of pepperoni and lifted it gingerly off the front of the ensemble that had taken them nearly an hour to mix and match in Claire's walk-in wardrobe.

Claire checked her own untouched slice of pizza, gripped casually between her fingertips, well away from her own nails (forty-five minutes). With her free hand she brushed invisible crumbs off her own outfit (seventeen minutes, Feb. *Cosmo*, Page 63).

She glanced at her reflection in Amanda's sunglasses. Hair okay, face okay, still not sure about the lip gloss. It was the same colour as the cabanossi on the pizza.

One of the hatchback guys glanced over. Claire and Amanda froze.

Claire suddenly realized that during all these weeks she'd never thought what she'd do with the pizza if one of the blokes actually came over to them. No way she'd eat it. Holding it was bad enough. Still, you had to look as though you had a reason for leaning against the pizza shop wall every Saturday afternoon.

She casually turned her head away from the boys so she was looking down past the video shop, the paper shop, the hairdresser and the other video shop.

To a small figure coming towards them. Hair ablaze in the sunlight. Glasses glinting. Cheeks pink and perspiring. Little brother.

'Oh puke,' muttered Claire.

Amanda looked round, saw Ben and glanced hopefully across at the hatchback worshippers.

'Perhaps he knows these guys,' she said without moving her lips.

'Only on a babysitter/client basis.'

Ben stopped in front of the girls. He stared at Claire's slice of pizza. Claire glared back.

'One word . . .' she said threateningly.

'Can I ask you something?' said Ben.

'Only if it doesn't involve money,' said Claire, relieved that the little dobber didn't seem to be taking advantage of his very strong blackmail position.

Ben looked through his sister's lush black fringe of lashes into her eyes.

'I've asked Mum and Dad but they won't give me a straight answer.'

Claire and Amanda froze, all but their eyes, which darted across at the boys, then met anxiously above Ben's head.

Amanda muttered through clenched teeth.

'Please, not here, don't ask where babies come from here.'

24

One of the boys looked over. The girls writhed with embarrassment.

Claire dropped her slice of pizza, pulled two dollars from her bag, thrust it into Ben's hand and pushed him away.

'Go. Go. Rack off,' she hissed.

Ben thought of trying his question anyway. Then he looked at the girls, who were studying the sky and the ground and trying to look as though they wouldn't notice if someone dropped a hundred megaton warhead on the blokes across the road. He decided not to.

He walked away slowly, stepping over Claire's slice of pizza. Questions burned inside him fiercer than any pepperoni.

He knew they'd cause just as much pain when they came out.

4

SPARE RIBS

Ron sat in the small, dingy office at the back of one of his shops and looked at all the paper.

The mountain of invoices on his desk, the sheaves of delivery dockets pinned to the board, the rows of ledgers on the shelves, the numerous abattoir calendars around the walls with their naked women segmented by dotted lines into Forequarters, Topside and Rump.

He was meant to be in meat, not paper.

These days it was other blokes who got to nick the baby fat off sweet-smelling legs of lamb and slice through heavy, marbled rumps with knives so sharp you could lop a finger off and not notice till you tried to give a rude sign to a bus driver on the way home.

But not for much longer.

Once the wholesale side was up and running he'd be able to afford an accountant on staff who'd rip through all this paper like a leaf mulcher.

Then he'd really be able to get cracking on expanding the business. Until one day the supermarkets wouldn't be able to touch him.

Wearily he grabbed the next invoice and

started checking the figures. He decided the accountant would be a woman so she'd get rid of those bloody awful calendars.

The office door crashed open and Wal, the manager of the shop, a big, cheery man in a bloodstained apron, came in carrying the morning's takings in a calico bag.

'Missed the plane to Rio again,' grinned Wal and dumped the bag on the desk.

Ron smiled. Wal made him smile.

Wal frowned.

'Jeez mate, you look pooped,' he said, his big happy face sagging with concern.

Ron rubbed the grey bags under his eyes.

'Got a lot on my mind,' he said. 'Getting the bulkstore open by next month mostly.'

'At least you won't have to bone and trim nights in Woolies to pay for this one,' said Wal fondly. 'Remember the second shop?'

Wal sat on the corner of the desk. The desk groaned.

'Ever thought, mate,' said Wal, 'if you sold the business now, this arvo, you could go to the beach with nearly a million cans of beer. And still have enough left over for an Esky.'

Ron smiled again.

'Million tinnies doesn't go far these days,' he said. 'Not when you've got a family.' He rubbed his hands wearily over his face.

'Wal,' he said, 'do your kids ever ask you questions you can't answer?'

Wal grinned. 'All the time. What's the capital

of Spain? Forty-seven minus ninety-three? It's just a phase they go through.'

Ron looked at Wal.

'Know what Ben asked me this morning? Why are so many people in the world starving?'

Wal thought for a moment.

'Curly one,' he said. 'Still, could have been worse. Guess what my Daryl asked me once? Where does the picture go when you turn the TV off?'

Both men laughed. Then they stopped. Wal frowned.

'Where does it go?'

Ron dragged himself out of the car and plodded wearily up the driveway. In front of him the big house sat solid and immovable under the starry sky.

He wished he felt solid and immovable.

He fumbled with his keys, closed the front door behind him, dumped his briefcase on the hall table, felt his way to the foot of the stairs and switched the light on.

And nearly jumped out of his skin.

'Ben!'

Ben sat on the third stair looking at him, the pile of magazines on his pyjama'd knees.

'Can I talk to you now, Dad?' he said.

Ron's shoulders sagged.

'Not tonight, mate,' he mumbled wearily. 'It's nearly midnight. Some other time, eh?'

He ruffled Ben's hair, stepped past him and plodded up the stairs, hoping with his last glimmer of energy he wasn't being a bad parent.

Suddenly he felt a jab of anger. Why should he be expected to worry about the world? Nobody in India gave a stuff that an Australian butcher had just spent Saturday afternoon and evening stuck in an office sweating over figures.

He stopped, turned and looked down at Ben.

'Anyway, you should be in bed.' He went upstairs to dream of paper.

Ben sat on his stair with the world's problems on his knees and a heavy heart.

Why won't Dad talk to me! he wondered. Sure he's busy but you can always find a moment. That's why I sat up half the night risking acne from lack of sleep.

He remembered other times he'd desperately needed to talk to Dad. Sitting up on the stairs had always worked then. Like the time Shane Moore had kicked the pedal off his bike on purpose and he'd desperately needed to discuss his plan to superglue him to the council garbage truck.

That night he and Dad had talked almost till dawn.

So why won't he talk now? wondered Ben. Perhaps it's me. He checked his breath. Perhaps I'm adopted and he's scared he'll blurt it out. Perhaps I've got cancer and he can only control his grief by not talking to me.

Ben tried not to think about these possibilities or about the world's problems. Maybe then they'd go away. Well, it seemed to work for Dad.

Monday morning. The local tennis courts were alive with women in white. Several thousand dollars worth of imported racquets flashed in the sun. Dozens of small, round objects moved in a blur.

Not balls. Tongues.

Di and her friend Jean had it down to an art. They swiped the ball back at their doubles opponents without a falter in the flow of the conversation.

Jean could actually time her forehand to stress a key word in a statement.

'You mean (whack) starkers?'

Di was worried.

'There she was on the front cover in all her glory and Ben didn't seem the slightest bit interested.'

She threw up a backhand lob and looked across at Jean.

'He should be at twelve, shouldn't he?'

Jean didn't take her eyes off the approaching ball.

'Jason is,' she said. 'Obsessed. Caught him peeking at me in the shower the other day. I was (whack) furious.'

She sent her forehand return hurtling past the two women chatting at the other end of the court.

'Well, I had this crummy old shower cap on, no makeup . . .'

Jean always played tennis with one hand holding her hair in place. She had evolved her own unique serving style. Racquet between the knees, toss the ball in the air with the racquet hand, grab the racquet and whack, over the net.

'The only thing Ben's obsessed with at the moment is the starving millions,' said Di gloomily.

'Never mind. Could be worse,' called Jean, getting into position for an approaching back-spin lob.

'Jason had a craze on earthworms. Dozens of the things wriggling round the backyard. Barry was (whack) furious. They can weaken the root structure of the lawn and bring down the value of the whole house. We had to have the entire garden sprayed.'

Ben pushed through the yelling throngs of school-uniformed Space Killers, video movie blackmarketeers and Aussie test teams.

In front of him Rev. Harvey's suede jacket receded across the playground. (With Rev. Harvey in it, of course. Miracles were thin on the

31

ground in state schools, much to Rev. Harvey's disappointment. A scripture teacher's suede jacket strolling unoccupied across the playground would at least take the little horrors' minds off the rude bits in the Bible.)

Ben put on a spurt and came up alongside Rev. Harvey.

'Sir . . . did you think of an answer to my question, sir?'

Rev. Harvey, a young man with straight hair, glanced around. No escape. No Hand of God to pluck him up and drop him into his car.

Without breaking his stride he put an arm round Ben's shoulder. Ben had to slip into a trot to keep up.

'I like to think of it this way, Ben,' said Rev. Harvey. 'If there were no starving people, how would we know to give thanks for our own full bellies? If there was no torture, how could we truly appreciate the heavenly gift of a quiet evening in front of the television?'

Ben wished they were in any part of the world where the chances of Rev. Harvey stepping on a mine would be greater than they were now.

'If there was no arsenal of nuclear weapons,' continued Rev. Harvey, 'poised to wipe out all life on earth, how could we be truly grateful for God's promise of eternal life in heaven? Eternal Life, Ben, Time Without End (beep beep beep) . . .'

Rev. Harvey took his arm from around Ben

and switched his digital watch alarm off.

'You'll have to excuse me Ben, I'm running late.'

He strode off into the carpark.

Ben realized the bell had gone.

The Space Killers, video movie blackmarketeers and Aussie test teams were all back behind their desks waiting to hear about River Capture on Sandstone Belts.

Ben watched Rev. Harvey's car pull out of the carpark. So much for religion, he thought. Three years in a row I've made a dill of myself in his nativity play, plus I'm allergic to straw, and when you need them they piss off to get a McDonald's.

Ben decided this Christmas he was going to offer his services to Mr Bright's production of The Rocky Horror Show.

He walked slowly back across the playground, alone.

That night at dinner Ben ate his beef curry and felt something burning inside him that had nothing at all to do with the effect of curry powder.

Ben looked at his father.

Across the table Ron chewed slowly, his mind elsewhere.

Ben looked at his mother.

Di was glaring at Claire, trying to get her

attention without Ron seeing. Claire was staring defiantly at the wall, her heaped plate of curry untouched in front of her.

Finally Claire glanced at her mother and Di signalled angrily with her eyes for her to eat. With an exaggerated gesture Claire picked up a single grain of rice, put it in her mouth and chewed vigorously.

Di glared at her.

Ron looked up and wearily watched the silent battle of wills in progress.

Suddenly he reached over and picked up the *National Geographic* from the sideboard. He held it open in front of Claire.

'Do you want to end up looking like this?' he said.

Claire looked at the photo of the stick-thin Ethiopian and tried to stop herself giggling but couldn't.

To their surprise, Ron and Di found themselves giggling too. They saw Ben looking at them stony-faced, but even with that they couldn't stop.

Ron nudged Ben across the table.

'It's only a joke,' he said.

Ben didn't smile.

So that was why they wouldn't talk about it. Only a joke. People starving to death and the world about to be burnt to a crisp and it's only a joke.

How could they?

Ben swallowed a mouthful of curry and it felt

like ice as it slid through his pounding chest.

He knew now exactly what the Feeling was, and what he was going to have to do about it.

5

NO CHICKEN

Ron smiled contentedly.

The sky was blue, the sun was warm, his pool was sparkling clean and all around him people were doing something that gladdened his heart.

Eating meat.

He threw a couple more steaks onto the sandstone-block gas barbeque and brandished his flashing steel in the hazy blue smoke like a Samurai warrior. One that didn't mind being seen in public in a paper chef's hat and a plastic Boss Of The Barbie apron.

Di moved among the guests with garlic bread. Everyone took some and juggled it along with their drinks and steaks against their New Season Leisurewear Pastels.

The only person to have viewed this idyllic backyard gathering with more contentment than Ron would have been a manufacturer of Instant Pre-Wash Stain-Remover.

The guests, women trim and tanned; men pale, overweight and tired; chatted, laughed and tore into steaks and people not present with equal gusto.

Di wandered over to Ron and slipped her arm

under his apron and round to where she could give his paunch a loving squeeze.

'Taking your mind off things?' she said.

'Haven't used the word wholesale all afternoon,' lied Ron grinning.

She gave him a big, wet kiss.

Jean, dressed more for a wedding than for a backyard barbie, came over with her husband Barry.

'Only thing about this wholesale meat caper,' said Barry loudly, 'the abattoir out the back here's going to ruin our property values.'

Everyone within earshot laughed. Ron pretended to prod Barry with the barbeque fork.

'I suggest we all sell up now and move to a better area,' continued Barry, 'like Calcutta.'

Everyone fell about. Barry was known as a bit of a wag up both sides of the street as far as his place.

Jean took Di to one side.

'How's Ben?' she asked. 'Through his phase yet?'

Di wrinkled her forehead.

'I think so,' she said. 'He seems a lot better lately.'

In the bathroom Ben stood in his underpants listening to the laughter and chatter filtering up from the garden below.

He heard Barry yelling, 'Phase . . . what

37

phase?'

In front of him in their rack were Ron and Di's His'n'Hers Electric Shavers.

He pulled one of the plugs out of the double socket and looked at the three shiny brass pins.

He ran his fingertip over the three tiny slits in the plastic facing of the socket.

Now the time had come he was scared.

Down in the garden Barry had just been re-minded about Ben's 'phase'.

'Starving millions?' He rolled his eyes. 'Where do they get them from?'

He tucked his drink under his arm, balanced his paper plate on one hand and put his other arm round Di.

'Di, take it from an old hand, phases pass. Or as in the case of our earthworms, pass on. Mind you, you might have to get Rentokil to spray Africa, India and Kampuchea . . .'

In the bathroom Ben listened to Barry's monologue, distant but crystal clear.

He heard a faint ripple of laughter and knew then he was going to do it.

But if he could hear them, then they might be able to hear him. He didn't want them to hear him. Not till it was finished. He had to use a silent method.

He pulled open the drawer below the sink and rummaged through old mascara bottles and half empty packets of Aspro.

Ah, there it was, Dad's old razor and yes, a packet of razor blades.

Barry's audience had gradually drifted away as usually happens at barbeques when someone drones on about the same subject for nearly fifteen minutes.

But Barry didn't seem to have noticed and kept on churning out the words between mouthfuls of steak to whoever was listening.

Which was Jean because she was loyal to her husband even though sometimes she wished someone would cement his mouth over, and Di because she was loyal to Jean.

'. . . the thing you've got to ask yourself about the Starving Millions is, has charity made them soft?'

Barry stuffed a chunk of steak into his mouth and chewed it into submission.

'I mean,' he continued, 'if I knew there were vast organizations running doorknocks and telethons all over the world with the sole aim of putting a bowl of curried prawns in my hands I'd think twice about going to work too. I don't say I'd necessarily lie around in the backyard and let flies crawl up my nose . . .'

He didn't notice that Jean was looking past him and gasping with horror.

Di followed her gaze and looked for a moment as though she would faint.

Oblivious, Barry put another piece of steak into his mouth. Then he noticed the sudden silence and saw that everyone else was staring aghast at something behind him.

Slowly he turned.

What he saw drained the blood from his face and froze every muscle in his body.

Standing close to him was Ben, naked except for his glasses and a white loincloth, his skin stained brown from his bare feet to his gleaming, shaven scalp.

The boy looked steadily at the ashen-faced man.

Barry tried to swallow his half-chewed lump of steak.

'In the time it takes for that mouthful of steak to reach your stomach,' said Ben softly, 'ninety people will die of hunger.'

Barry stopped swallowing and started to choke.

The guests gaped.

The lettuce slid unheeded off Claire and Amanda's plates.

The only person to move was Jason, a cheery-faced boy of Ben's age. He hurried towards Ben to get a closer look.

'Fancy dress. Ripper.'

Jean, his mother, grabbed him and pulled him back as if from the brink of a cliff.

Ron and Di stared at their son, dumbstruck.

They stared at his brown skin. They stared at the white cotton tablecloth knotted round his waist and between his legs.

They stared at the shiny, bald dome of his head.

They realized they had a problem.

6

LASHINGS OF TONGUE

'Why?'

Ben sat on the edge of the settee in the lounge-room. A towel had been placed between his dark brown skin and the light brown leather. His loincloth was beginning to cut off the circulation in his upper legs.

'Just tell me why?'

Ron spoke with the exaggerated softness and slowness of a man about to go through the roof.

He and Di stood looking down at their small brown son. Outside the evening breeze blew paper cups across the empty yard.

Ben looked up at their grim faces.

He wished he could say a magic word and in a flash of laser light get really big muscles and a bullet-proof cape and fly with a parent under each arm to the African villages he'd seen on TV, and the South American government torture chambers he'd read about, and the big concrete basements in Russia and America where men older than the ones who'd dribbled at Grandpa's funeral brunch sat ready to fire bombs that would make whole countries as shrivelled and mottled as the skin on their shaking hands.

'Because,' he said quietly, 'I don't understand why nobody gives a stuff about what's happening.'

'Don't you use that language . . .' said Ron, his voice rising dangerously, his face going red.

Di grabbed his arm and spoke with exaggerated calmness.

'We're going to be civilized about this,' she said to Ben. 'Despite the fact that you broke up our barbeque, upset our friends, used nearly a whole tube of my instant tan lotion, none of us is going to lose our temper.'

Ron lost his temper.

He advanced on the cowering Mr Alsop, his face the colour of rump steak.

'Your job is to teach geography,' he screamed, 'not inflame impressionable young minds with propaganda!'

Mr Alsop, a pale young man who at that moment wished he'd taken the geology elective at college so he could now be drilling for uranium in the middle of the Simpson Desert, retreated.

He backed across the classroom, banging into desks and knocking chairs over until he came up against the blackboard with a jolt.

'Mr Guthrie, please,' he pleaded, 'I've done nothing of the sort. All we've done this year are

Tropical Zones and Tundra. Haven't we, Ben?'

He looked pleadingly at Ben, who stood pink-skinned and smooth-domed by the door in his school uniform.

'Don't forget, sir,' said Ben sweetly, 'our excursion to study the weather systems over the Sydney Cricket Ground during the Second Test.'

Mr Alsop smiled nervously at Ron.

'Famine and Starvation isn't until Year Eleven,' he said, and hastily added, 'even then it's an elective unit, interchangeable with Temperate Ski Zones II.'

He flung a piece of chalk at the window, where a dozen faces ducked down out of sight.

Word had already swept the playground that Guthrie's dad was laying into Alswap for letting Guthrie catch leukaemia on the cricket excursion.

The air in the Guthrie bathroom was thick with pre-work and school urgency and the smell of burnt toast.

Claire sat on the toilet brushing her teeth with an electric toothbrush, the toothpaste in her ensuite having run out.

Ron stood in front of the mirror with a towel round his waist, running his electric shaver over his tired face.

Next to him Di had one foot up on the sink,

shaving her leg with a safety razor.

Ben wandered in in his pyjamas, rubbing his eyes. He took Di's electric razor from its rack, flicked it on and guided it across his bald scalp.

Ron and Di looked at each other.

Di said it first.

'I think we need some help.'

The psychiatrist sat in her chair and looked at Ben sitting in his.

She was a large, middle-aged woman who smelt like she'd fallen into a tanker of Chanel No 5 a couple of years earlier.

She looked thoughtful.

Eeeeeeaaaaauuuuuoooowwwww.

Behind her a workman was drilling holes into the office wall with a power drill.

A large oil painting of a green and purple cat with six heads, lying on what appeared to be a rice salad, leant against the wall waiting to be hung.

'Ben,' said the psychiatrist. 'If you had to sum up all your feelings about the world's problems in one sentence, what would it be?'

Ben thought for a moment. The workman drilled on. Ben wondered if the psychiatrist was deaf. He was going to be history if he had to do this in sign language.

'How can we just carry on as if nothing's wrong?' he said.

The psychiatrist thought about this for several minutes filled with the noise of drilling. White dust settled on her hair.

Ben tried desperately to think of the sign for 'How'.

At last she spoke.

'What exactly do you mean by wrong . . .?' She spat out a small piece of wall plaster. 'Do you mean wrong in the Jungian sense of an absence of rightness or do you subscribe to the Reichian theory of the inversion of moral criteria?'

She wrinkled her brow and muttered to herself.

'Or have I got that wrong?'

Di sat anxiously in the waiting room flicking through a magazine and trying not to look at the young man in the corner taking pencils one by one out of a box and smelling them.

Next to her Ron hammered away on his calculator, papers from his open briefcase spread over the coffee table.

The door opened and the psychiatrist came out of her office with her arm round Ben.

Ron and Di stood up.

'Well, Mum and Dad,' said the psychiatrist heartily, 'we've given the fat a good old chew and I don't think you need worry any more. I think we've managed to screw a few lightbulbs into a few sockets.'

Di glanced at Ron with relief.

The psychiatrist looked down at Ben.

'What do you say Ben, ready to rejoin the land of the living?'

Ben shrugged apologetically to his parents.

The young man in the corner never knew if the bald kid was apologizing for his misbehaviour or for the psychiatrist's performance.

7

DRIPPING

Ron steered the Motor Vessel 'Cutlet Queen' into the secluded, tree-shaded inlet and breathed a sigh of relief. His precious cargo was safely at its destination.

Not that the Harbour had been choppy, but you couldn't be too careful when your precious cargo was the manager of the second largest abattoir in New South Wales and his charming wife.

'What an utterly superb spot,' said the Abattoir Manager's charming wife.

'Utterly,' said Di, just a shade too loudly. 'The first time we saw it we said "This is utterly, utterly superb".'

Ron flashed her a warning look, which he changed to a warm smile as he turned to face his guests.

'We always picnic here when we're on the boat,' he said with what he hoped was exactly the right amount of casual self-confidence for a soon-to-be successful wholesaler.

While Ron steered the cruiser towards the little sandy beach and dropped anchor, Di topped up the Abattoir Manager's champagne and his wife's gin and low calorie tonic.

She opened the big hamper and handed round seafood canapes.

'Oh goody,' said the Abattoir Manager's wife, 'I love little bits of prawn on biscuit.'

Di fleetingly weighed Ron's business future against the pleasure of pushing the Abattoir Manager's wife overboard and ramming her.

She told herself to calm down. It was just this thing she'd always had about women with huge sunhats and mouths big enough to store them in.

The Abattoir Manager ate, drank, smacked his lips and looked around with the deep feeling of excitement felt by all folk born west of Dubbo when confronted by more than three litres of water in the one place at the one time.

He slapped Ron on the back expansively. Ron glowed, partly because he sensed his business future falling into place, partly because he'd caught the sun.

'Well, Ron,' said the Abattoir Manager, 'if you can promise doing business with Guthrie Wholesale Meats will always be this enjoyable, I think my abattoir can come up with the right goods at the right price.'

Ron squeezed Di's hand without the others seeing.

The Abattoir Manager's wife licked prawn juice from her ring-encrusted fingers.

'But only if you promise not to tell another soul about this divine spot,' she said, swinging her arm vaguely around and slopping gin and low calorie tonic onto her husband's Hawaiian shirt. 'Two minutes and it'd be swarming with grotty little families in rowboats.'

Ron squeezed Di's hand again, this time harder to warn her against carrying the Abattoir Manager's wife below decks and chopping her up for bait.

'We've been all over the world ,' continued the Abattoir Manager's wife, 'inspecting abattoirs, Greek Islands, Fiji, The Bahamas – this beats the lot. So utterly cut off from all the cares of the arggghhhhhhh!'

She gave a long, horrible, bloodcurdling scream, dropping her gin and tonic and bit of prawn on biscuit and pointing to the water near the boat.

Floating there was what looked like a bale of cloth, roughly human-sized.

'My God,' said the Abattoir Manager, 'it looks like a body.'

It was a body.

Face down, head submerged, it was clad in some sort of rough cotton. It bobbed gently next to the boat.

'Quick Clarrie, that hook on a pole there.'

The Abattoir Manager's wife wrestled the boathook out of its clamps. Her husband helped her.

The wash from the rocking 'Cutlet Queen' caused the body to half roll in the water. Ron and Di caught a glimpse of a scuba tank strapped to the body's chest, then a flash of something else round and smooth.

Di felt all the blood in her body run into her feet.

Ron felt a flash of pain behind his eyes. For a moment he thought his guests had accidently swung the boathook through the back of his skull. The something round and smooth was Ben's bald head.

'I'll kill that kid,' he muttered under his breath.

The Abattoir Manager and his wife leant over the side of the boat and lunged at the body with the boathook. The boat rocked wildly and the wash turned the body over.

Ben's pink domed face looked up at them. His eyes quickly closed.

The Abattoir Manager and his wife managed to get the hook through the thick cloth wrapped around Ben and started hauling him aboard.

'He's still alive!' screamed the Abattoir Manager's wife.

Ron grabbed at the boathook.

'Leave him in there,' he yelled.

Di buried her face in her hands.

The Abattoir Manager and his wife looked at each other in horror.

'I don't believe it,' mouthed the Abattoir Manager's wife.

The Abattoir Manager pushed Ron away and hauled Ben onto the deck with the hook.

Ben slid off the hook and flopped down on

his back, dripping. A large soggy hessian poncho covered most of his body. The bulge of the air tank made him look like a wet monk.

The Abattoir Manager tore the air valve out of Ben's mouth. Ben spluttered and coughed and opened his eyes and looked at them.

'He's alive. Thank God,' said the Abattoir Manager.

His wife turned angrily to Ron and Di.

'No thanks to you,' she said. 'You'd have left him in there to die. The fish had already eaten his hair.'

'You don't understand,' said Di. 'He's our son.'

The Abattoir Manager stared at Ron in horror. He struggled to find words.

'I . . . I . . . I . . .'

Ron struggled to find words to explain.

'He . . . we . . . I . . .'

The Abattoir Manager's wife exploded with righteous anger.

'I don't believe it! I just do not believe it!'

Di buried her face in her hands again.

Ben sat up and tried to address the assembly. He'd swallowed what felt like several litres of seawater and it kept bubbling out of his mouth as he tried to speak.

'In the time it took you to haul me in . . .'

'I . . . I . . . I . . .'

'He . . . we . . . I . . .'

'Incredible. Absolutely incredible.'

'. . . the mutilated bodies of eight political

prisoners . . .'

'You . . . you . . . you . . .'

'We . . . he . . . we . . .'

'Of all the selfish, irresponsible . . .'

'. . . were found floating in South American rivers.'

'He . . . we . . . he . . .'

'In South American rivers,' repeated Ben.

No one was looking at him.

'. . . heartless, callous, brutish . . .'

The Abattoir Manager finally found the words. He fixed Ron with a thunderous brow.

'Some people are not fit to be parents,' he growled, adding darkly, 'or businessmen.'

8

NOT MUCH CHOP

Ben sat on the edge of the bath while Di wrapped him in a big, warm, soft, fluffy towel and bawled at him.

'. . . you could have drowned, you could have caught pneumonia, you could have drifted into the propeller and . . .'

She stopped and turned away.

Ben felt a surge of elation. They'd got the message. All this pneumonia stuff was just Mum trying to cope with it.

He remembered when he'd first read about political torture in South America. He hadn't been able to stop eating waffles and icecream for two days.

Ron came in to the bathroom and started washing the winch grease off his hands.

Di looked at him in exasperation.

'Well, say something,' she said.

'Forty cents a kilo extra I had to offer him,' said Ron, 'and half a gallon of Chanel for his wife. I was that close to losing the contract.'

Di closed her eyes for a moment, then spoke softly.

'Okay Ben, this has gone far enough.'

She pointed to her sewing-room curtains lying in a heap in the bath looking less than happy in their new role as a soggy poncho.

'Those'll come out of your pocket money.'

What pocket money, thought Ben.

'We've stopped his pocket money,' said Ron.

'Well, we'll start it again,' said Di.'And these are going under lock and key.'

She snatched the His'n'Hers Electric Shavers from their wall-rack.

'And starting tomorrow,' she said, crouching down in front of Ben, 'I drive you to school, I pick you up, and the rest of the time you spend in your room.'

She pulled the towel tightly around Ben's shoulders.

Ben looked up at his grim-faced parents, a small, pink, bald, bespectacled face peering happily out from the folds of the towel.

'You can chain my body,' he said, 'but you can't chain my mind.'

On the TV screen Hiroshima lay in ruins, the once-thriving Japanese city looking to Ben like a team of men with sledgehammers had smashed every upright object into rubble and dust and splinters and then carted away most of the debris.

And all the people.

'They do that with models,' said Jason cheerfully. He was sitting on Ben's bed staring at the screen in fascination and rhythmically transferring the contents of a box of chips into his mouth.

'I saw it on "The Making of Star Wars",' he crunched.

A sombre voice narrated over the scenes of bleak devastation.

'. . . within two kilometres of the nuclear blast people are vapourized instantly. It is beyond two kilometres that the true horror begins . . .'

Jason stared at the hideously burned people with their misshapen features and huge open sores.

'That makeup's lousy,' he said. 'Indiana Jones was heaps better. Anyway I'm sick of Making Ofs. It never looks as good as the actual movie.'

He hit 'off' on the remote control and turned to where Ben was shaving his head with an electric razor.

'What's it like?' he asked.

Ben blew expertly across the rotating heads of the razor.

'It works fine. You're sure your Dad won't miss it?'

'No way,' said Jason, 'he's got millions. I mean what's it like being mental?'

'I'm not,' said Ben matter of factly.

'That's one of the first signs,' said Jason seriously, 'thinking you're not. That and people making you stay in your room.'

Ben knew it wasn't Jason's fault. He had problem parents. They didn't have a clue. Brains like woodwork teachers.

Not like Mum and Dad. They were coming along very nicely. Okay, they weren't saving the world but at least they were worrying about it a bit.

'We've taken him to see people, we've tried punishment, discipline . . . I don't know what to do.'

Ron rubbed his hand wearily over his face.

'I've got to get security clearance to have a shave,' he said plaintively.

Wal brought his cleaver smashing down through the lamb carcass, removing a leg. Fortunately from the carcass.

'I'm no psychiatrist, Ron,' said Wal. He waggled his bloody cleaver and flashed an evil grin. 'Be a bit of a worry if I was . . . but I reckon he's doing it for the attention.'

He deprived the lamb of another leg.

'It's the age,' he said. 'When I was his age I used to walk into lamp-posts, just so's people'd look at me.'

'So what do I do?' asked Ron.

'Ignore it.' Wal put down his cleaver and wiped his hands on his apron. 'That's what we did with my sister's youngest. Kid went round claiming she could fly. We just ignored her.'

Ron felt a tinge of relief that he wasn't the only bloke with a weird kid.

'Did she stop?' he asked.

Wal looked at his old mate and employer.

'Yeah,' he said reassuringly. Then he remembered something.

'Now she reckons she's invisible.'

Di and Jean sat by the tennis court waiting for their doubles opponents to arrive.

Di stared at the hard green surface of the court. She'd just told her friend all about the boat incident but it hadn't made her feel any better.

Jean was deep in thought. She reached her verdict.

'He's just doing it for the attention,' she said, fluffing her hair and smiling at a good-looking young coach walking past.

'That's not like Ben,' said Di doubtfully.

'It's the age,' sighed Jean, watching the coach's bottom in its tight white shorts receding into the distance.

'Bit of hair they can sit on and they think they're Sylvester Stallone.'

Jean stared at the net.

'I just wish I knew the right way of handling it.' She thumped Jean even as her friend's suggestive smirk crossed her face.

'There is only one way,' said Jean, serious again. 'Ignore them. We've been ignoring Jason for ages now and it's worked like a dream. Not a peep out of him for months. Some of the performances we used to have. All that rigmarole about his tongue turning black after Barry had the garden sprayed . . . take it from me Di, ignore him.'

'At this stage I'll try anything,' said Di desperately. 'Okay, from now on we'll ignore him.'

9

COLD SHOULDER

Ron and Di sat at the dining table ignoring Ben.

It wasn't easy.

While they picked at T-bone steaks the size of doormats Ben, naked except for his loin cloth and tanning lotion, stared at them steadily from under his bald dome and slowly ate a small pile of rice from a wooden bowl.

Ron stared at the carpet, the sideboard and the ceiling.

'Ceiling's holding its colour well,' he said.

Inside Ben was holding his breath. He knew all this staring at the carpet, sideboard and ceiling was just a last desperate bid for escape before Dad broke down and sobbed about the state of the world.

Di stared at the ceiling, the sideboard and the carpet.

'So's the carpet,' she said.

Claire looked at them both as if they were stark raving mad.

'Have you two been hitting the bottle?' she asked incredulously.

'Be quiet,' said Di, 'and chew your lettuce properly.'

Di, Jean and a couple of their friends floated languidly in the pool on their inflatable chairs.

Above them an azure sky stretched away for ever, the sun caressed their bronzed bodies and the warm, fragrant air rustled the palms next to the patio.

Di trailed her hand through the cool water and sipped her drink. She needed just one thing to make this paradise.

No son floating face down among them wearing her sewing-room curtains, that's what she needed.

Not long now, thought Ben, hoping Mum wouldn't be up the deep end when the grief about the state of the world finally hit.

The other women studied their nails and bikini tops and pretended they couldn't hear the little bubbles from Ben's scuba tank popping at the surface.

Except for Jean.

She gave a big yawn, stretched, and nonchalantly put her glass on Ben's back as he floated past.

But then, thought Ben, she's done this sort of thing before.

'Just ignore him.'

The harassed mother pulled her child away from the ghastly apparition next to the Italian slingbacks on special.

The shoe shop was buzzing as the other customers whispered and shot disapproving glances at Di and Ben.

Di sat and stared straight ahead as if bringing a bald, loinclothed boy in to be fitted with football boots was the most normal thing in the world.

Her heart was pounding.

So was Ben's. How much longer could she keep this up?

The hapless sales assistant, who'd almost died at birth and now wished he had, crouched in front of them with a football boot in one hand and Ben's bare brown foot in the other.

'Football socks'd be best,' he said unhappily.

Di looked down with a air of vague surprise.

'Isn't he wearing them?' she said mildly. 'Oh, no, he's not.'

She reached into her bag and dropped a pair of Ben's football socks into the sales assistant's lap. She did a Jean yawn and stretch and smiled sweetly at the other women in the shop, who all quickly looked away. She felt sick.

The assistant slid the socks onto Ben's brown legs.

'St George supporter, eh?' he said doubtfully, wondering if they played footy in India.

He put a football boot on Ben's foot.

'Comfortable?' he asked.

Ben looked down at him.

'With forty thousand kids starving to death every day?' said Ben. 'Are you?'

The sales assistant looked at the gaping women.

He looked at Di, who was studying in minute detail the Italian slingbacks on special.

He wondered how she could be so calm.

Ben looked at her and wondered the same thing.

Di leapt for one of Jean's famed forehand returns and hammered it back over the net.

Sometimes she preferred playing singles. You didn't have to talk. Which made it easier not to think. Which when you were trying to ignore someone was a big help.

Except by thinking that she wasn't ignoring him. Bum.

She swept Jean's return back over the net.

She'd read once that Navratilova or one of the other top women players emptied her mind totally on the court.

Di tried to empty her mind totally.

Jean's lob bounced high in front of her and she swung and connected with the perfect centre of her racquet. The ball touched down just inside Jean's base line and cannoned into the fence, giving Di game and set.

Or would have done if it hadn't hit a large placard showing an orange nuclear explosion about a metre above the net.

Di turned away.

It was easy for Navratilova, she didn't have a son wearing a rubber joke-shop skull mask and one of her best French sheets daubed with 'Nuclear Madness' in luminous paint chained to the net holding up placards in the middle of the court.

She kept her back to Ben.

'I'm ignoring you,' she muttered through clenched teeth.

'I'm ignoring you.'

Cripes, thought Ben, sweating inside his rubber mask, I think she is.

'Don't eat it all at once.'

Wal handed the parcel of meat over the counter to the customer with a forced smile.

'I won't,' said the customer, giving Wal a forced smile back.

They were both trying to pretend that there wasn't a bald twelve-year-old boy in a loincloth sitting in the shop window in the centre of a display of chops and sausages.

But there was.

Ben stared past Wal and the customer to

where his parents stood in the doorway of Ron's office pretending not to look at him.

He took the string of sausages from round his neck. Perhaps he was too camouflaged. Perhaps they couldn't see him.

'Oh, my God,' said Di, turning away and biting her car keys.

'If the health inspector sees this he'll throw the book at me,' said Ron. His face was grey with fatigue. He glanced over his shoulder at Ben and saw a tall, angular woman of about fifty wearing a black coat come into the shop.

'Oh no, that's all I need,' he said. 'Mad Esmé.'

They're looking at her, thought Ben, why aren't they looking at me?

The woman started handing out leaflets to the customers waiting to be served. The customers, who normally ran a mile from women in black coats handing out leaflets, grabbed them voraciously.

Any reading matter to get their eyes off that mad kid in the window doing the pot roast impersonation.

Esmé went over to Ben, gave him a leaflet and a clenched fist salute of solidarity, and left the shop.

Ben looked at the leaflet. 'Save Their Skins', it said across the top in neat hand-lettering. And underneath, 'Anti Fur Slaughter Demo. Feldman Furs. Sat. 2pm'.

Ben folded the leaflet and tucked it inside his

loincloth. He had his own problems.

He continued his unwavering stare at Ron and Di.

Di lay awake, staring into the darkness of the bedroom. Next to her Ron lay motionless, his eyes closed.

'I can't take much more of this,' said Di.

Silence. Except for Ron's deep, slow breathing. Di gave him a nudge.

'I'm thirty-seven and I've got a bald son.'

Silence. She gave Ron another nudge.

'Ignore him,' said Ron without opening his eyes.

'You can't ignore something like that,' said Di, hearing a tiny note of hysteria creeping into her voice.

Ron opened his eyes and put his hand on Di's.

'Just hang on till next week,' he said. 'Once the bulkstore's open I'll have more time.'

Di felt anger tear through her like a fingernail through a pair of tights.

'For us or for the four more shops you're planning to open?' she snapped.

Then all she felt was limp and guilty.

'Why do you have to push yourself so hard Ron?' she said wearily. 'We've got everything we need. I don't even know why you're opening a wholesale bulkstore.'

Ron struggled up onto one elbow, incredulous.

'Half the world starving and she doesn't know why I want to provide for my family.'

He took his hand from hers, flopped back down and rolled over.

Di looked at his back. On the sheet covering him, faintly where it didn't quite wash out, was the word 'Madness'. Di nodded in agreement.

Ron lay with his eyes open, muttering through clenched teeth.

'I'm ignoring you. I'm ignoring you.'

He didn't mean Di.

He meant the brown figure hanging outside the bedroom window, the one with the noose round its neck and the sign clutched to its chest. 'Apartheid Victims.'

Outside Ben tried to ignore the chill night air and the hang-gliding harness cutting into him in forty-seven different places.

He opened his eyes and saw Dad looking at him.

He snapped his torch on and shone it on the sign.

He saw Dad close his eyes.

He saw the tiny, rhythmic movement of Dad's lips and knew what they were saying.

'I'm ignoring you . . . I'm ignoring you . . .'

Shit, thought Ben, he is.

10

VEAL MEAT AGAIN

The first day of the Subtle Method was Saturday.

Ben sauntered into the kitchen wearing jeans and a T-shirt and leafing idly through a World Health Organization Interim Report On Infant Mortality In The Third World.

He strolled over to Di, who was crouched by the microwave oven staring intently into it. Casually he allowed the report to fall open on the work bench.

'What's for lunch, Mum?' he asked brightly.

Di didn't take her eyes off the interior of the oven.

'Nothing if this thing doesn't go round,' she snapped. 'Grey pork.'

She thumped the side of the microwave.

Di wasn't the only thing about to blow a fuse in the kitchen that morning. Everything that plugged in was plugged in and whirring, blending, juicing, toasting, percolating, mixing and waffling fit to explode.

Ben slid the report closer to Di. She didn't look up. Ben stood and watched her.

The Subtle Method had come to Ben the

night before in the tree outside his parents' room.

As he'd hung there watching his father's lips move, he'd asked himself for the ninety-four millionth time How Can They Ignore What's Happening In The World?

Sure there was sex, and work, and tennis, but not day and night, twenty-four hours a day, week in week out, year after year.

Which was the amount of time they spent ignoring what was happening in the world.

Then an awful thought had struck him.

What if he was helping them to ignore it all?

By giving them something to take their minds off it?

Him?

Ben pushed the report closer to Di, who was still scowling into the microwave.

'Go round!' she yelled, giving the oven another thump. 'Go round!'

The Subtle Method was hitting them with hard, detailed information with no distracting factors like women with bare boobs or him in painted sheets.

He pushed the report still closer to Di, who had pulled open the microwave oven door and was trying to rotate the rotisserie by hand.

The Subtle Method had one drawback.

It was easy to miss.

Di burnt her hand on the roasting dish, swore and became aware of a huge bushfly crawling across the cupboard door in front of her.

She grabbed the report, rolled it up and whacked it against the cupboard door.

The rotisserie started to slowly revolve.

Di dropped the fly-spattered report back onto the bench.

Ben abandoned the Subtle Method.

Di closed the microwave oven door and the rotisserie stopped revolving.

Ben looked at Di.

Di looked at the microwave.

They stayed that way for a while.

Then Di swung round to face Ben in anger and exasperation.

'Okay! You win!' She snatched up the report and read from it in a loud garbled monotone. ' ". . . four out of five babies born in the third world will suffer from malnutrition. Two out of five babies die before reaching their fifth birthday . . ." Okay? Satisfied?' She flung down the report. 'Now for God's sake go out and get some exercise.'

For a few seconds Ben thought about how much exercise he'd get kicking the microwave round the block.

Then suddenly he remembered something.

'Can I go with Claire?' he asked.

Di saw Claire heading for the door with Amanda, both in their Saturday afternoon best.

'Claire, where are you going?' asked Di.

'I told you,' said Claire. 'Into the city. To the er . . .' She reddened and glanced at Amanda, who had just at that moment got something in her eye.

'. . . art gallery,' said Claire.

Di was in no mood for playing detective.

'Take Ben with you,' she said.

Claire looked horrified.

'Into the city?' she wailed. 'Oh no Mum, we can't take him into the city.' She pointed behind her cupped hand at Ben's bald head, pleading. 'Not like that'.

Di was unmoved.

'He goes or you stay.'

They went.

Although as they hurried along the crowded city street trying to keep a couple of steps in front of Ben they wished desperately they hadn't.

They just knew that once the big city sophisticates noticed Ben's head, all would be lost.

'Hey Julian, check the bald kid.'

'Strewth Jonathan, there's no way chicks from The City would hang around with a younger brother that looked like that. They must be from one of those daggy bush suburbs that hasn't even got its own record shop. Ho ho ho.'

Claire and Amanda needn't have worried. The shoppers trudged along with their eyes to the ground, concerned only with shopping and the likelihood of getting AIDS from contact with shop door handles.

No one poured ridicule on them.

What did happen was worse.

Claire and Amanda, with Ben close behind them, turned a corner and found themselves surrounded by leaping, chanting, drumming, robed, painted, shaven-headed Hare Krishnas.

The girls backed away, half-remembered Sunday paper headlines flashing through their heads.

'White Slave Drug Cult' . . . 'Moonie Kidnap Horror' . . . 'Does Meditation Cause Migraine?'

But the Hare Krishnas didn't carry them off for the white slave trade. Instead they saw Ben's bald head and gave him a cheerful thumbs up as they danced past.

Bit frivolous, thought Ben, all this dancing in the street. But as he turned to look again at the shaven-headed men in their robes his heart pounded and he felt he could soar up to the very tops of the tall buildings all around him. And poop on everyone.

Claire and Amanda wanted to sink into the pavement.

Failing that, they frogmarched Ben into the nearest chemist and emerged a few seconds later with him wearing a large straw hat.

'We could take him,' said Claire, racked with guilt. 'It'll be dark.'

'It's an R-rated movie,' said Amanda long-sufferingly. 'They won't let him in.'

Ben sat in his booth in the video arcade and

pulled his straw hat down over his ears so he wouldn't have to listen to the girls arguing over him. Surely Claire wasn't going to stuff it up now?

In the booths on either side, intergalactic wars were being won and lost. Ben looked at the screen in front of him. Armies of spaceships and monsters waited to be hurled into frenzied conflict by a silicon chip and a twenty cent piece.

Ben wondered if anyone had invented a Big Sister video game.

Mascara, Big Sister From The Slimy Deep, Locked In Mortal Combat With Amanda, Mutant Best Friend From A Lost Galaxy . . .

'It's only two hours and we'll be back . . .'

Claire was leaning over him, loading a milkshake, a packet of chips, an ice cream and a bag of lollies into his lap.

'. . . When I was your age I'd have killed for all this.' She swept her arm around the arcade. 'Okay?'

She took three steps away and three steps back.

'You'll be okay?'

'I'll be fine,' said Ben. 'Go on, hurry up, you'll miss it. Bye.' Phew, close escape.

He grasped the video controls like a boy about to do battle in farthest reaches of deepest

73

space. Until, glancing out of the corner of his eye, he saw that Amanda had dragged Claire away.

Then he took off his straw hat, dumped the chips and stuff into it and pulled from his pocket the leaflet he'd been given in the butcher's shop window.

'Save Their Skins. Anti Fur Slaughter Demo. Feldman Furs. Sat. 2pm.'

As he read the address pencilled across the bottom he tingled with excitement. Then he climbed out of the booth and headed for the exit, dropping the goody-filled hat into the arms of a startled ten-year-old Space Mercenary.

11

MUTTON AND LAMB

Ben heard the chanting even before the fur shop was in sight.

'Out! Out! Out! Out!'

By now the tingle was a cold sweat. His first demonstration. He'd seen old news film of the Anti-Vietnam demos of the seventies, tens of thousands of people thronging the streets, arms linked, chanting, singing. A sea of humanity surging with a shared cause.

Ben turned the corner.

In the doorway of the fur shop stood two people.

One was Esmé, the tall woman in the black coat who'd given him the leaflet in his father's shop. She was trying to reason in a clear, calm voice with the furious manager of the fur shop, who was pointing to the deserted street and shouting.

'. . . Out! Out! Out! . . .'

'. . . but nylon fur is just as warm,' Esmé was saying. 'You could at least give your customers the choice . . .'

For a moment Ben thought the veins in the fur shop manager's neck would burst clean through his starched white collar and pink bow tie.

'That's obscene,' he grimaced.

As Ben got closer he could hear the tinkle of glasses and the chatter of voices coming from inside the shop. A couple of hawk-faced women with ski tans peered out through the door, saw Esmé, smirked to each other and disappeared back inside.

A sign in the shop window announced 'New Season Parade – 2pm'.

'Look, you old ratbag,' yelled the manager at Esmé, pointing back at the shop, 'one foot in there again and I'm calling the police.'

He stormed back into the shop and shut the door.

Ben watched as Esmé pulled a roll of tape and a large sign from her cane shopping bag and stuck it over the one in the window. The new sign read 'Their Deaths Are On Your Shoulders'.

As she smoothed down the tape, she noticed Ben standing watching her. She looked at him for a moment thoughtfully.

'I remember you. Six fifty a kilo.'

For some reason her voice reminded Ben of their family doctor. Perhaps she smoked a pipe as well.

'Is it over?' asked Ben.

Esmé rattled the locked shop door, picked up her bag and signalled for Ben to walk with her.

'Saturdays are never much good,' she said

ruefully.

'Were you the only one who turned up?' said Ben. He couldn't believe it. There wasn't a train strike or anything.

Esmé, who'd been looking at him with amused interest, transferred her gaze to the pavement for a few seconds.

'What have you done to your head?' she asked.

They walked in silence for a few more seconds.

'It's to remind people that if you don't have enough to eat your hair falls out,' said Ben.

He'd hesitated because everyone else he'd said that to had taken it the wrong way. Claire had thought he was having a go at her diet. Ron had taken it as a dig at his thinning scalp.

Esmé was impressed.

'I see,' she said in a way that showed she realized this was no ordinary run-of-the-mill bald twelve year old.

She touched her own thick grey hair, cut into a rough pageboy style around her long face.

'I think I'll stick to posters,' she said. 'Won't be a minute.'

And with that she darted into a milkbar. Ben followed her in.

On the counter was a hot food bar with three chickens turning slowly on a spit and several more already roasted sitting under hot lamps.

Esmé pulled a poster out of her bag, unrolled it and stuck it to the counter below the hot glass.

It was a photo of a fridge with a trickle of blood coming from the freezer compartment.

Ben read the caption.

'That Chicken In Your Freezer Has More Room Now Than It Did When It Was Alive.'

Good one, he thought. People have much bigger freezers than they really need.

The milkbar proprietor, a middle-aged Italian man, put down his newspaper.

'Yes?'

From behind the counter he couldn't see the poster. Esmé pointed to one of the roast chickens.

'Do you know,' she said softly, 'that that chicken has more room now than it did when it was alive?'

The proprietor frowned. He wasn't quite sure if he'd heard right.

'You want a chicken? Four ninety-nine.'

'Have you ever thought,' said Esmé, 'about what those chickens suffered?'

The proprietor caught her drift, or thought he did.

'They're not stuffered,' he said patiently, 'they're barbeque. Four ninety-nine.'

Esmé continued with quiet determination.

'About the misery they suffered in the horrible confinement of the battery farm . . .'

Ben saw it dawn on the proprietor that something was going on.

'Four ninety-nine or nick off,' said the proprietor with a suspicious frown.

'You don't have to buy chickens that have been tortured in tiny cages,' continued Esmé in her quiet, forceful voice. 'You can buy free range chickens that have roamed around . . .'

'That's right,' said Ben, trying to work out what all this had to do with big freezers.

The proprietor looked over the counter, saw the poster, dashed round from behind the counter and grabbed Esmé by her coat collar.

'That's it,' he shouted, 'I'm calling the cops. You want a free chicken, you'll get one in jail.'

Ben realized Esmé was in trouble.

He began to cough and wheeze and make himself go red in the face. He tugged at Esmé's coat.

'Mum,' he croaked, 'I'm having another asthma attack.' And he turned on a fit of hissing and wheezing that made the Espresso machine on the counter feel quite inferior.

Now that Esmé had been elevated to the sacred ranks of motherhood, the proprietor let go of her collar and backed away.

Ben grabbed her hand and pulled her out of the shop and into the street.

Esmé fired a parting salvo over her shoulder.

'Be careful, my son's a solicitor.'

The proprietor was having second thoughts about Esmé as a mama. He made a traditional Sicilian gesture beseeching her to stick a sheep's head up her bum.

'What did you mean about chickens being tortured?' asked Ben as they walked away.

79

Esmé looked at him in surprise.

'In battery farms, crammed into tiny cages from birth, filled with chemicals . . . you know,' she said.

'No,' said Ben.

Esmé stopped.

'Where did you think chickens came from?' she asked.

'The supermarket,' said Ben.

She strode off down the street, leaving Ben standing bewildered.

She beckoned him to follow her.

12

HAM AND EGGS

Ben hobbled off the bus on the balls of his feet, legs numb after sitting in the same position for an hour and a half. He tried to look ready to spring into action.

But there wasn't a tortured chicken in sight.

Just scrappy paddocks on both sides of the road behind carbon-monoxide choked trees. There was a cow. But it was on a hoarding advertising hamburgers.

The bus growled away leaving a haze of foul smelling exhaust.

Esmé started climbing over a rusty wire fence.

'Like all prisons,' she said, 'they always stick chicken farms miles from the nearest bus stop. Come on.'

Ben and Esmé trudged across a paddock whose occupants were a couple of lethargic horses, contemplating their futures on the backs of stamps, and a few rusting car bodies.

Ben had always liked the country, that big, clean place at the end of the expressway. Dad had taken a weekend off once and they'd gone in the car.

Must have been counting motorbikes while we were passing this bit, thought Ben. Even the Australia II Memorial Reserve at home leaves this for dead and it's got drinking fountains in the shape of winged keels.

After more trudging they reached a huge corrugated iron shed. Esmé swung herself over another fence and pulled Ben over. She crept towards the door of the shed.

Ben followed, realizing he didn't have a clue what they were actually going to do.

He saw that the door was chained and padlocked shut. His pulse dropped to very high. It couldn't be anything too drastic.

Yes it could. Esmé took a pair of boltcutters from her cane shopping bag and sliced through the chain with a practised grunt.

She turned to Ben.

'Okay, we free as many of the poor blighters as we can.'

She pushed the door open. What had been merely the sound of several thousand chickens muffled by corrugated iron now became a roar of clucking.

Ben found his legs wouldn't move.

Esmé saw him hesitating.

'Look,' she said gently, 'just pretend this is the first day you walked into class with that hairdo.'

Ben followed her inside.

It took his eyes a while to get used to the gloom, so for the first few seconds he was blinded and deafened. Then he found himself looking at thousands and thousands of chickens in tiny wire cages, stacked from floor to roof, stretching away into the distance.

He remembered the Old MacDonald's Farm picture book he'd had as a kid. One page sprang to mind, a farmyard filled with fat white hens pecking the earth.

These miserable creatures were from a different planet.

He walked down an aisle, horrified. The lank, greasy feathers. The deformed beaks. The sores. The dull, hormone-bloated eyes. And the deafening noise of misery.

Under each cage was a chute leading to a conveyor belt which in turn led to big egg-sorting machines. Next to one of these Ben picked up an egg box from a stack waiting to be filled. On the lid were the words 'Fresh Farm Eggs' with a drawing of a traditional farmyard.

Suddenly the squawks near Ben got even louder. He spun round.

Esmé had opened a cage door and hauled out a chicken, which was trying for the first time in its life to walk.

'Come on,' she yelled, 'pull your finger out.'

Ben watched the chicken stagger on its knees for a bit more, then realized Esmé was talking to him.

He pulled open the door of a cage and thrust his hands in, trying to get a grip on the scrawny, flapping bird inside.

The cage wasn't any bigger than the average Kentucky Fried Chicken box but he couldn't get hold of anything solid to hang onto.

As the chicken scrabbled in a frenzy and feathers dropped out of its already patchy wings, Ben felt he was going to be sick.

Esmé, who had a dozen cages open, the squawking birds fluttering and limping around her, came over and took him by the arm.

'Go and keep a look out,' she said.

Ben ran out into the sunlight and leant against the hot corrugated iron wall of the shed, gasping in huge lungfuls of air.

After being in there, out here was paradise. He looked across the green fields and trees.

And saw a white car hurtling along the dusty approach road. A white car with a badge on the door!

He banged frantically on the wall and yelled in through the doorway.

'Someone's coming!'

All Ben could see was a mass of chickens hysterical with freedom. Esmé's voice echoed out.

'About time. I rang them an hour ago.'

Ben couldn't believe it. Rang the police? He'd heard of police informers but never one who'd dobbed herself.

Ben turned as the car skidded to a stop and two men leapt out, one wearing a brown suit and carrying a microphone, the other in a T-shirt with a portable camera on his shoulder.

Ben looked again at the badge on the car door. It was the logo of a TV station.

'Why do we always get the animal stories?' muttered the cameraman.

'Don't knock it,' said the reporter, checking his hair in the wing mirror, 'she's good value.'

Several chickens fluttered out of the shed door and Esmé appeared with several more in her arms. She waited till the red light went on on the camera, then threw the chickens into the air with a dramatic gesture.

The cameraman zoomed into her. Her hair was full of feathers and her face and coat were streaked with droppings.

Then Ben heard a siren.

Another car hurtled round the bend in the approach road, this time with a blue light flashing on the roof.

'Run for it!' yelled Ben. 'The cops!'

'You buggers,' Esmé said to the reporter and cameraman. 'You promised.'

She ran back inside the shed.

Ben followed her. Behind him he heard the reporter calling them back out, pleading that the video camera wouldn't work in the dark.

Ben ducked down behind a row of cages as the police car screeched to a halt outside.

Esmé was flinging open cage doors as fast as she could, leaving the chickens to find their own way out.

Two burly cops stepped into the shed and went for Esmé.

'Okay, you've got no right to be here, lady,' announced one of them.

An egg splattered onto his chest.

'I'm here in the name of humanity,' shouted Esmé and hurled another egg. The policeman whipped his cap off and used it as a shield. Or omelette bowl.

He advanced on Esmé through a barrage of eggs and grabbed her in a bear hug.

Ben stood up.

'Leave her alone,' he yelled.

The other policeman sprinted towards him. Ben looked around frantically. No eggs! A million egg-laying chooks and he chooses constipation row.

He turned and sprinted down the aisle.

'Come here, grandad,' said a gruff voice close behind him.

The young constable peered through the gloom at the small, bald figure running in front of him.

He threw himself into a flying tackle and the two of them crashed onto a pile of bulging, revolting-smelling sacks.

'Got you, you old bastard,' grunted the constable.

He turned Ben over and his policemanly face crumpled with surprise.

Then it went very stern again.

13

CHILLED PORK

Di and Ron sat in the living-room, their faces taut with worry, trying not to look at the pine clock on the wall.

Five minutes to seven.

Ron picked up some papers and ran his eyes down the columns but 'lamb' and 'beef' might have been messages from some distant galaxy for all the sense they made to him.

Di tried to run through in her mind the angry scene they'd had when Claire arrived home alone, the accusations, the tears, Claire's vow to stay on a hunger strike till Ben turned up . . . Di couldn't concentrate.

Four minutes to seven.

At seven o'clock they were going to have to accept that their twelve-year-old son was missing, that something terrible might have happened to him, and that they were going to have to ask the authorities to supply them with the awful details.

Di tried to count the number of years she'd lived in fear of that, the ring at the door, the two grim-faced figures in blue, 'Mrs Guthrie?', caps in hand as if already at a funeral . . .

The door-bell rang.

They leapt up and flung themselves into the hallway. Ron got the front door open.

Ben stood there, the porch light shining on his dirt-streaked face. Mud stuck to his jeans and T-shirt. A chicken feather floated down onto the tiles.

Di and Ron buckled with relief.

'Where have you been?'

'Claire's been home for hours.'

'Why didn't you ring?'

'Another five minutes and we were going to call the police.'

The police, in the form of two muddy constables, stepped forward out of the shadows and stood, grim-faced, on either side of Ben.

Ron and Di stared at them in alarm.

'Mr and Mrs Guthrie?' said one of the policemen. 'I'm Constable Mulock and this is Constable Harris. We'd like to come in to investigate some serious allegations that have been brought to our notice.'

They took Ben's arms and guided him past his horrified parents into the house.

'Cripes, Wayne, he's right. The nuclear equivalent of forty-seven tons of TNT for every man, woman and child on earth.'

The two policemen stood in Ben's room, poring over the magazine Ben held open for them on his desk. They looked deeply worried.

'I thought he was exaggerating,' said Constable Harris.

'It gets worse,' said Ben. He turned the page gravely. Inside he was jumping for joy. What a day. First Esmé, now the cops. People who cared.

He looked at Ron and Di, who were standing open-mouthed in the doorway, their horror mingled with utter amazement.

They're not bad people, he thought. If the cops can do it, they can. They just need time.

Constable Mulock picked the magazine up and read from it, his flat courtroom voice tinged with alarm.

' "If just twenty per cent of known nuclear weapons were detonated, human life would cease to exist in the northern hemisphere . . ." '

The two policemen looked at each other.

Constable Harris' voice wavered as he spoke.

'Makes parking in a bus zone seem a bit irrelevant, doesn't it?'

Wal swept his arm expansively around the truck loading bay.

'. . . and this is where the meat'll be loaded for the shops.'

Jean and Barry stared intently at the truck loading bay, nodding thoughtfully. The trouble with guided tours of wholesale meat bulkstores was that there wasn't much you could say. 'I like the colours' worked well in art galleries but the bulkstore was basically grey. 'It doesn't look six hundred years old' was great in museums but the bulkstore had only been finished on Tuesday. Bulkstores sort of restricted you to things like 'it's very nice.'

'It's very nice,' said Jean.

Barry kept nodding. He wasn't really sure why they were there. Sure it was Ron's pride and joy but they'd be at the official opening on Monday. He had better things to do than traipse through freezers and cool rooms while a fat butcher waffled on about thermostats and offal chillers and Ron and Di tagged along behind looking glum.

'That's it,' said Wal proudly. He turned to Ron. 'Well mate, couple of days and you'll be up there with the big boys.'

Ron didn't look as though this prospect set his major organs aquiver, in fact he didn't look as though he'd even heard what Wal had said.

Ron glanced at Di, who was looking similarly dour. He cleared his throat.

'Actually . . . Di and I didn't ask you here just for the tour.'

'It's Ben,' said Di.

'We've tried everything,' said Ron. 'Discipline, psychiatry, ignoring him . . . and he ends up on TV being chased by the police.'

'Terrible.' Wal shook his head, his normally jolly face grieving. 'I was watching World of

90

Disney and I missed it.'

'You're our best friends,' said Di, 'and we need your advice about what to do next.'

She looked imploringly at Wal, Jean and Barry.

'Electric shock treatment,' said Barry.

Jean glared at him.

'I've seen it all before,' he continued, 'young blokes shave their heads, next thing they've got tattoos . . .'

Jean stepped forward, grinding her heel into Barry's foot and laying her hand on Di's arm.

'Perhaps he just needs something to take his mind off this obsession with major world problems,' she said. 'Something closer to home.'

'When Daryl was picking his spots,' said Wal, 'we bought him boxing gloves.'

Di looked intently at Jean.

'You mean a problem closer to home for him to worry about?' she asked.

'Plummeting property values,' said Barry, massaging his foot.

Ron took Jean's arm urgently.

'You mean a problem within the family?'

'I don't just mean a problem,' said Jean, 'I mean a disaster.'

Ron and Di stared at her.

14

MINCING WORDS

Ben was glad to see Dad had dressed for the occasion this time.

He remembered the last time they'd sat together on his floor for a chat. The sight of the seams in Ron's safari suit stressed beyond the previously known tolerance for poly-cotton weave had made it hard to concentrate on the matter in hand.

This time Dad was much more sensibly dressed in a loose-fitting tracksuit with plenty of give in it. Its seams were in the peak of condition, this being only the second time Dad had worn it since Mum gave it to him for Christmas four years ago.

But he still didn't seem to be comfortable. In fact while Ben spoke, Dad wriggled and writhed and looked like a man who wished he was somewhere else.

'. . . so after nuclear war in the northern hemisphere thirty percent of the ozone layer in the southern hemisphere would be destroyed.'

'Um . . . Ben . . .'

Ben saw that his father was trying to interrupt him. Here we go, he thought. The Birds

And The Bushflies Episode Two. Well, I'm going to get this out. Some things are more important than what mummies and daddies do together when they love each other very much.

'It's the ozone that protects us from the sun,' he continued urgently, stressing the words with his hands.

'Ben . . .' said Ron.

'Everyone in Australia would be blinded,' shouted Ben.

'Ben . . . um . . . look mate, I'm afraid I've got some bad news too.'

My God, thought Ben, this man's capacity for evading the obvious is without limit. Is there anything he wouldn't do to avoid having to face facts?

Ben wondered why cross thoughts always came out in headmaster talk.

'It's . . . er . . . your mother,' said Ron.

'Mum?'

'It's just been discovered that . . .' Ron swallowed. 'She's not well, Ben.'

Ben felt a flicker of panic dancing around inside him.

'Not well?'

'It's a rare neuro-metabolic condition.' Ron was staring hard at the carpet. He looked up at Ben.

'It's not serious so long as she has plenty of rest and doesn't have to worry about things.'

He lifted his hand to ruffle Ben's hair, realized you can't ruffle a smooth dome, and patted

Ben awkwardly on the shoulder instead.

Ben didn't notice.

'Can't they cure it?' he demanded, panic creeping up his throat. 'Those vast, highly-trained organizations you're always on about. Hospitals . . . specialists . . .'

Ron squirmed unhappily.

'Er . . . they haven't seen anything like it before.' He took a deep breath. 'All they know is she's very fragile and if she has too much stress or worry about . . . well, chicken farms or . . . or ozone levels . . .'

Ron took another deep breath.

'. . . Well, she didn't want me to tell you this but she could . . . she could . . .'

Ben saw from the misery on Ron's face what he was trying to say.

He leapt to his feet, his heart pounding, the room behaving like something out of a bad rock clip.

'Mum!'

He had to find her. He ran out of the room.

Ron dragged himself painfully to his feet, calling after his distraught son.

'Ben, she's very fragile.'

Di thundered across the court and smashed a high-velocity return over the net and past her bewildered opponent.

Jean, sitting on the sideline, applauded and

went back to fiddling with the sunglasses in her hair.

Di skipped back to the base line to receive the next serve, continuing her conversation with Jean as she went.

'It'll have to be me,' she called out, 'if we want to get it done this year.'

The woman at the other end served and Di hammered the ball back.

'You know where Ron's mind is most of the time,' she continued, 'if I leave it up to him . . .'

Jean signalled frantically to Di to be quiet because running towards them, his face heavy with concern, was Ben.

But Di was away, sprinting across the court to fling herself at a backhand return.

Ben stopped and gripped onto the wire safety fence, panting hard. He stared at his mother as she leapt around lunging and volleying, his concern gradually giving way to amazement. Fragile? She was leaping around like John McEnroe.

Di smashed a set-clincher past her opponent and noticed Jean pointing discreetly across the court. She turned, saw Ben and came over to him.

'Hi love,' she said with a sad little smile. 'I was hoping to see you 'cause I want to have a little word with you.'

She pointed to the gate at the end of the court and they started walking towards it, the fence between them.

Ben's heart was pounding. Please, please don't let the little word be rare neuro-metabolic condition. He prayed that Di would now reveal there'd been a mix-up at the lab, a careless technician confusing her blood sample with that of a ninety-year-old alcoholic snake handler. Anything that she not be sick.

'It's about Dad,' said Di. 'Now I don't want you to worry but we've just heard he's got a bit of a problem with his liver.'

Ben stared at his mother through the wire fence, his fear gradually being replaced by a horrible, cold suspicion.

'And kidneys,' said Di. 'Now it's nothing to worry about as long as he takes it easy and doesn't get worked up . . .'

They reached the gate. Di opened it and put her hands on Ben's shoulders.

'. . . but there is a tiny danger that if he has a shock, say from seeing you on TV again, or too much stress, say from hearing about nuclear war or something, he could . . . well, there is a chance he could . . .'

Before she could say the awful word Jean rushed over and started tugging frantically at her tennis dress. Di looked up. Galloping to- wards them across the carpark, red-faced and gesticulating wildly, was Ron.

Ben looked at his approaching father and then at his mother's horrified face. His sus- picion was very quickly becoming anger.

It had all been a lie. Everything. The rare

neuro-metabolic condition. The liver and kidneys. Dad's concern about superglueing Shane
Moore to the council garbage truck. Everything.

Di tried to save the situation.

'There's nothing actually wrong with his
heart,' she stammered, as Ron lumbered towards them. 'Exercise is fine, in fact the doctor
said for liver and kidney problems exercise is
the best . . .'

She saw from Ben's face that they'd blown it.

Ron staggered up to them, gasping for
breath.

'We agreed I'd do it,' hissed Di.

'Only if I couldn't find an opportunity,'
gasped Ron.

Jean buried her face in her hands, cringing at
the sheer volume of her friends' incompetence.

'Liars!' screamed Ben, and turned and ran,
his eyes filling with tears. He didn't want to
think or feel, just run.

Ron and Di clung to each other, rooted to the
spot with shame and guilt.

'Ben!'

'Ben!'

15

ONE MAN'S MEAT

It was the first block of flats Ben had been inside in his life and he was trying to knock them down.

Or at least the door of number forty-seven.

His tears had dried on the train trip out to the grimy industrial suburb and been replaced by an ice-cold determination to do what he was now doing.

As he stood there on the bleak landing, pounding on the door's cracked paintwork, he knew exactly why his parents didn't give a stuff about what was happening to the world.

Under those familiar outsides they were evil, scheming, selfish, lying monsters with green scales and little red eyes and waxed black moustaches.

A hand fell on his shoulder.

He spun around.

Esmé was looking at him thoughtfully.

'How did you get my address?' she asked.

Ben saw the faint marks on her black coat where the chicken droppings hadn't quite washed out.

'I heard you giving it to the police.'

'Pity you couldn't have made this much racket on that occasion,' she said dryly. 'Might have saved me the inconvenience of an appearance in court.'

'What did they . . .?'

'Suspended sentence. Next time they'll put me in the slammer with the chooks. That's if they catch me.' She gave a grin.

'I want to come and live with you,' said Ben.

Esmé's grin faded.

'Really,' she said dryly.

'I want to help you free chickens.'

'Indeed.' Her voice made the Simpson Desert seem like a lake.

'I can be a better lookout,' said Ben eagerly. He turned to the door and started pounding on it and yelling.

'They're coming! They're coming!'

Esmé hurriedly pulled him away from her crumbling paintwork.

'Very good,' she said. 'What about the starving millions?'

'We can help them in our holidays,' said Ben. 'Take overseas trips.'

'And what do your parents think of that little arrangement?'

Ben stared out across the industrial landscape. On the horizon, pipes towering above an oil refinery spewed flames into the sky. Ben wondered if the pipes were wide enough to stuff parents down.

'They don't care,' he mumbled. 'They're

selfish liars.'

'That's as maybe,' replied Esmé, her voice softening a little, 'but what do they think of their son becoming an apprentice chicken commando and part-time Son of God?'

She drew a halo in the air above Ben's bald head.

'Dad wouldn't even notice I'd gone,' said Ben bitterly. 'All he cares about is opening his stupid wholesale meat store tomorrow.'

Suddenly he felt he had to prove to Esmé he wasn't part of Ron's animal slaughtering empire.

'I'm getting better at it, watch.' He threw himself at the front door and battered at it, yelling at the top of his voice.

'The police are coming! The police are coming!'

Along the landing, doors flew open and anxious residents peered out. Esmé hurriedly stuck her key into the lock and bundled Ben inside.

'Last time anyone yelled that out around here six of my neighbours threw their TV sets over the back balcony.' She closed the door behind them.

Ben didn't hear her.

He was staring, appalled, at Esmé's flat.

It was a single room about the size of his bedroom at home but that's where the similarity ended. This one had a tiny kitchenette crammed into one corner and another corner partitioned off with sheets of frosted glass. It was dark and smelt of stale bread.

Ben counted five pieces of furniture. A table with a faded pink laminex top, a straight-backed wooden chair with a cracked vinyl seat, an armchair with a blanket thrown over it to stop the springs sticking through, a wooden reading lamp with a fringed shade, and a mattress on the floor.

For a fleeting moment Ben thought she'd been burgled and this was just the junk not worth taking. But the sight of Esmé unconcernedly throwing her coat over the back of the chair and whistling while she filled the kettle made that unlikely.

'You live . . . here?' he said. He realized it was a pretty stupid thing to say but he couldn't help it.

'Only during the week,' said Esmé sarcastically. 'I have a mansion in the south of France for weekends.'

Ben wandered around the room in a kind of shock. He stared at the walls, which were bare except for a couple of Animal Liberation posters. He stared at the plastic washing basket full of shoes and books on the floor by the mattress. He stared at the few clothes on wire hangers. And the length of string they hung from tied between the window frame and a pipe on the wall. He stared at the lino on the floor.

'Where's the carpet?' he said.

'Cup of tea?' asked Esmé.

Ben stared at the mattress on the floor, its sheets neatly folded back and tucked in under a nylon sleeping bag opened out for a quilt.

'Where are the legs off your bed?'

'They ran off together,' said Esmé. 'Cup or yoghurt pot?' She held up a china cup with no handle and a plastic yoghurt pot with most of the colour scrubbed off.

'Do you live just in this one room?' asked Ben, knowing she must do but hoping he'd missed something like a breakfast room out the back and maybe a rumpus room.

'Don't look so shocked,' said Esmé, amused by the furrowed brow under his shiny smooth dome. 'If this was Calcutta there'd be two families in here. Empty this for me.' She held out a battered blue metal teapot.

Ben stepped over to the kitchenette and surveyed the scanty fittings. The funny curved fridge. The portable plug-in hotplate. He couldn't see the microwave. The one at home was off being fixed half the time too.

He took the teapot and went to empty it into the sink.

'Not in the sink,' said Esmé.

'It's okay,' he said, 'Hungry Henry . . .'

'Who's Hungry Henry?'

Ben had never heard anyone over three ask that before.

'The automatic waste disposal,' he said pointing to the plughole in the sink. The plughole which didn't have an automatic waste

102

disposal.

Ben looked at Esmé.

'Wouldn't you rather have a real house?' he asked.

'I've got better things to do with my money,' she said, pointing to a poster like the one she'd stuck to the hot food bar in the chicken shop.

That's ridiculous, thought Ben. Those posters can't cost that much. He noticed for the first time that Esmé wasn't wearing a single bit of makeup.

'But you could spend a bit more on yourself.'

It was Esmé's turn to look serious.

'How could I?' she said. She picked up a can. 'My tea.'

Ben read the label. Vegetarian sausages. He'd never heard of vegetarian sausages. Perhaps they were made from animals who were vegetarians.

'The cost of this can is my busfare to a farm where I could save fifty chickens.'

'Why did you buy it?' asked Ben.

'I didn't. I pinched it.'

Ben stared at her. Was this what you had to do if you cared about the world? He looked around the room again. If this was Calcutta there might be two families living there but they'd have a TV and a carpet and legs on the bed.

'So,' said Esmé, 'when are you moving in?'

Ben didn't know what to say.

Esmé came over and put her arm round him.

'You can do much more good at home,' she said softly.

16

LIVE AND LOIN

Ben lay awake in bed wondering if he was as bad as his parents.

He sat up, switched on his bedside lamp, climbed out of bed, dragged the mattress off the bed base onto the carpet and lay down on it.

He tried to relax. The furniture loomed above him.

It felt strange.

It felt awful.

He stood up and dragged the mattress back onto the base.

Then he lay down and looked around.

He wondered if he could live without a pine bed base, a carpet, a wardrobe with sort of slits in the doors and a full-length mirror inside, a desk with a yellow top and built-in moulded plastic pencil holder, a video recorder, a custom-made pine TV trolley on castors, hand-printed curtains from Finland or Iceland or somewhere, an angle-poise desk lamp with dimmer and self-reflecting globe . . .

He didn't think he could.

Did this mean he didn't care either?

He heard a noise outside the door, switched

the bedside lamp off and pretended to be asleep, his eyes closed and his mind seething.

The bedroom door opened slowly and Di crept in holding her dressing gown around her. She switched on the bedside lamp and sat on the corner of Ben's bed.

Ben opened his eyes and looked at her.

'Heard you bumping around,' she said softly. 'I couldn't sleep either. Dad and I just want to say sorry.'

Ben turned away violently and closed his eyes.

'We're not as bad as you think,' she continued. 'People change, that's all. Other things become important. Like you.'

She leant forward and kissed him on the side of the head. There was a pause. Then he heard her get up and quietly leave the room. The door clicked shut behind her.

He opened his eyes. Lying next to his head on the pillow was a photograph. He held it under the light.

It was black and white, grainy, faded, and it showed a group of people sitting round a camp fire at night. Ben studied it closely. A woman was playing a guitar and a couple of the people were holding placards with strange signs on them, like clocks with four hands that were saying five o'clock and six o'clock and seven o'clock at the same time.

Ben remembered where he'd seen those signs before. At school in history when they did

The Sixties. All the pictures of demonstrations and rock concerts had them. They meant Ban The Bomb.

There was another placard being held up by someone in the group. Ben squinted to make out the blurred lettering. 'Butchers For Peace.'

Then he saw the face under the placard.

It was thinner, smoother, with greasy slicked-back hair and it was much younger than Ben had ever seen it.

But there was no mistaking it.

It was Dad.

Ron hurried to the garage looking tired and tense. This wasn't unusual, most mornings leaving for work he looked tired and tense.

It was just this morning he looked worse.

The greyness from under his eyes seemed to have run in the shower and spread over most of his face. Including his lips.

He heaved his briefcase into the car and flopped in after it. Just as he was about to turn the ignition key he saw out of the corner of his eye something move towards him out of the shadows.

This was it. He'd heard rumours this sort of thing went on but had never believed it. Hired muscle from the Mr Bigs of meat wholesaling. 'Just a word of advice, Mister Guthrie. It's a very crowded line of business what you're trying to crack into. If you get our drift.' Broken legs. And not the ones in his shop window.

He scrabbled for the lock buttons on the doors.

Then he saw it was Ben.

'Dad, can I have a word?' shouted Ben through the glass.

Ron wound down the window.

'Not now, mate,' he said wearily. 'I've got a million things to do for the opening this arvo. Tonight, eh?'

He turned the ignition key and drove out of the garage and down the driveway.

Ben stood watching the departing car.

'Why did you stop?' he yelled.

He looked down at the photo in his hand.

Butchers For Peace.

17

STUFFED HEART

'The big day,' said Wal. 'Here's to Ron.'

'To Ron.'

Di and Jean clinked their champagne glasses with Barry and Claire.

Across the inside of the bulkstore roof was strung a huge banner saying 'Grand Opening' and underneath it stood groups of people holding glasses and nibbling delicacies on Jatz biscuits.

They were mostly employees from Ron's shops or senior meat industry types. You could tell Ron's employees, they had an almost noticeable air of excitement in their chatter and only a hundred and ninety-seven fingers and thumbs between the twenty of them.

The senior meat industry types wore striped ties and contrary to Ron's moment of paranoia that morning wouldn't have considered breaking his legs in a million years. Just drinking all his champagne in twenty minutes.

'Hang in there, mate,' said Wal cheerfully, raising his glass as Ron hurried past. Ron just about managed a smile. If he'd looked tired and tense that morning he now looked double tired and triple tense.

'He was awake all night worrying,' said Di to Jean.

'About Ben?'

'About the wholesale price of mutton.' That was a slight exaggeration but Di was still feeling a bit resentful. She'd wanted Ron to come with her into Ben's room. Digging out the old photo had been a flash of inspiration but it had really needed flesh and blood back-up. Still, 'once the bulk store's open' had been Ron's regular cry so he wouldn't have any excuse after today.

'Where is Ben?' asked Jean.

'Went off on his bike this morning,' said Di. 'Thank God he's getting some exercise. Might even meet some girls.' Well, you could hope.

'You know what they say,' said Wal. For some reason he'd marked the occasion by putting on a shirt one size too small and was having trouble getting a soothing finger down between his neck and the collar. 'Exercise makes the heart grow fonder.'

Nobody was sure if this was a joke or not and there was a brief awkward silence until Barry saved the day by being tactless.

'So we won't be seeing a performance by the Domed Crusader.'

Jean would have kicked him but the shoes she'd put on to match her Spring Carnival racing hat were killing her.

Ben wouldn't do anything today, thought Di for the hundredth time. Not today. He

110

wouldn't. He'd had the photo with him when he'd left the house that morning so it must have made an impression. She felt better.

'Excuse me, Ladies and Gentlemen.'

Ron was standing in front of the red ribbon stretched across the cold room doors. He was holding his arms in the air.

'Excuse me . . .'

'Bit of hush, please,' yelled Wal, and when the hubbub had died down and everyone had turned to face Ron, 'Speech! Speech!'

There was a patter of applause and Ron stared down as if he'd only just noticed the floor in his new bulkstore was concrete. Then he looked up at the expectant faces and took a deep breath.

'I don't want to make a big speech here today . . .'

One of the apprentices gave a low cheer and a couple of his mates tittered. Di wondered if butchers ever slipped and cut their own heads off.

'. . . we all know why we're here and . . . I just want to say it's been a hard slog but we've made it and . . .'

Ron paused, breathing hard.

Come on, thought Di, you rehearsed it enough times in the shower. God, he looked grey.

'. . . and I want to thank my staff for their hard work and my family for their understanding and support.'

Di relaxed and smiled and applauded with the others.

Ron slipped his hand into his pocket and brought out her sewing scissors.

'I hereby declare Guthrie Wholesale Meats open for business.'

They all applauded again and he turned and cut the ribbon.

The cold room doors slid open.

Inside hung a row of beef carcasses with red ribbons tied to their back legs. But it wasn't at these that the assembled onlookers gasped with shock and amazement.

It was at the small bald boy hanging from a hook by the collar of his jacket holding a blow-up of a photo of a campfire and looking steadily at Ron.

Ron saw the stunned expressions on the faces in front of him and turned back to the carcasses.

He saw Ben.

Di watched in horror.

Ben opened his mouth to deliver his carefully rehearsed plea but instead watched helplessly as Ron gasped for breath, clutched at his chest and collapsed.

The thought flashed through Ben's mind that this was more acting but he saw his mother scream and the guests yell for somebody to get an ambulance and he saw his father's face twisted in agony and he knew it was really happening.

'Dad!' he yelled. 'Dad!'

He tried desperately to get down to where Ron lay gasping and groping at his shirt front but the meat hook had pierced his collar as deeply as the pains that were stabbing into Ron's heart.

Then Ron stopped gasping and lay still.

'Dad!' screamed Ben, 'Dad!'

18

TALKING TURKEY

Ron didn't die.

Wal gave him the kiss of life and thumped his chest which restarted his heart. It was a supreme act of friendship from a man who at no stage in his life had even remotely considered kissing another bloke.

Then the ambulance arrived, by which time Ben had been lifted sobbing from his hook and held tightly, together with the wailing Claire, to Di's pounding ribcage.

They bundled Ron into the back of the ambulance with an oxygen mask over his face and plugged him into a shelf of monitoring equipment. Then they sped through the streets, siren screaming, Di, Claire and Ben huddled in the back clinging to each other and Ron's hands.

Nothing Ben had ever seen on a television screen had filled him with as much dread and terror as that little wavy green line flickering across the tiny screen of the heart monitor.

At the hospital there was an extra moment of panic when a group of orderlies slid Ron, still connected to the monitor, out of the ambulance onto a trolley and ran away with him.

But Di and Claire and Ben gave chase down brightly lit corridors to where they stood now, in an intensive care ward, looking at Ron lying in an oxygen tent surrounded by banks of beeping, flashing equipment.

Ron lay there, still and grey, his only signs of life electronic ones.

One of the doctors came over to them.

'There's a very good chance that if his condition continues to stabilize and we don't experience any adverse trends towards deterioration he'll be okay,' she said. She gave a smile and squeezed Di's arm.

But they could see from a glance exchanged between the other two doctors that it had been a close thing.

And still was.

Ben looked at his father and knew that if it was in his power to sacrifice the lives of a thousand people in another part of the world so that Ron would open his eyes and climb out of the plastic tent and hug them all and drive them home he'd do it

Ten thousand.

A million.

It was his fault.

He looked up at his mother and gripped her hand tighter.

'I just wanted Dad to start caring again,' he said. 'You can't just stop caring.' He let go of her hand. 'Can you?'

'It's not your fault,' said Di softly, stroking

his bald head.

She struggled not to show the fear she was feeling.

'Let's hope he's learnt his lesson,' she said, looking at Ron.

'. . . no . . . no . . . Wal, listen, you can get a better price than that . . .'

Ron heaved himself up onto one elbow with difficulty, cursing nurses who tucked the sheets in too tight and the electrodes still taped to his chest which almost ripped the skin off him if he moved more than six inches.

His face was still pale and tired, nowhere near as pink as the stuff that had him gripping the receiver with frustration.

'Lamb's on the way down,Wal. Hold out . . . Call their bluff . . .'

He heard voices outside the door, hung up and stuffed the phone under the bedclothes. His pulse was up, he could hear it beeping away on the 747 flight deck next to the bed.

That was one way to get out of this place and back to running the business he thought as he tried to breathe slowly and steadily.

Fly yourself out.

The door opened and Di and Ben came in.

'Ben!' cried Ron delightedly. 'You finally made it.'

It took Ron several seconds to realize what

was different.

Ben's hair.

A blond fuzz covered his entire scalp.

Stack me, thought Ron, with the jeans and T-shirt and, well it's virtually a crew cut, he looks like a normal kid.

Ben walked over to the bed and stood looking at Ron.

It had flashed through his mind in the lift coming up that his fantasy a week ago in intensive care had come true. A million people had died in other parts of the world.

But Dad's recovery hadn't depended on it so he didn't care. All he cared about at the moment was . . .

'Dad,' he said softly, 'I'm sorry I gave you a heart attack.'

Ron felt something in his rib cage cavity that had nothing to do with heart attacks or electrodes ripping out his chest hairs.

He leant forward and put his arms round his son.

'Ben, don't be silly,' he said, shocked.

Di bent over and kissed him on the cheek.

'I've tried to explain to him,' she said with an edge to her voice, 'that you had a heart attack because you abused your body for years and years with far too much work and not enough exercise and relaxation. Isn't that right?'

Ron let go of Ben and looked up at him. He wanted desperately to put Ben out of his misery but a bloke couldn't in all honesty agree to something that exaggerated.

'Ah . . .' he said, '. . . well . . .' He wriggled awkwardly.

A doctor breezed into the room.

'I'm sorry,' he said with a briskness that may not have been meant as a joke, 'the patient mustn't have any difficult questions. Just easy stuff like who's going to win the test.'

He turned a knob on one of the pieces of monitoring equipment and the room filled with the 'beep beep' of a steady heartbeat.

'Still,' said the doctor turning the volume down a bit, 'for a week after stalling the motor you're sounding pretty good.'

Di looked at Ron and her eyes glowed.

The doctor looked at Ron and his eyes narrowed.

He stepped over to the bed and pulled the phone from under the covers.

'And if you take it easy,' he said, giving Ron a long hard look, 'you might just stay that way. Otherwise we'll all be up to our armpits in blood and gristle.'

'You can't scare me,' said Ron, 'I'm a butcher.'

The doctor stopped at the door.

'That reminds me,' he said, 'don't eat so much meat.'

He swept out.

'He can't scare you,' said Di, 'because you're a stubborn fool.'

Ron blew her a kiss. Then he beckoned Ben to come back to the bedside. Ben went over.

'Mate,' said Ron, staring at the sheet as if he'd never seen a phone come out of a bed before, 'when I was coming round after the . . . after the scare, there was one thing that kept nagging at the back of my mind.'

An alarm bell went off in a ward corridors away.

Ron looked at the ceiling and continued.

'Something I chickened out of. Ben . . . if there's anything you want to ask about . . .' he looked Ben in the eyes, '. . . anything in the world, fire away.'

Another alarm bell went off. This time it was inside Di.

No, thought Di, not the Starving Millions. Please, not now.

Ben looked at his father steadily for a long time. Two desires took shape inside him. I want to keep Dad safe and I want to make him happy. Ben knew that if the first was to happen, the second wouldn't always be possible. So he took the opportunity to make Ron happy now.

'Dad, where do babies come from? I mean, is it actually the ovary or the endometrium?'

Di mentally hugged Ben.

Ron looked around in alarm. Babies? Endometrium? What about the Starving Millions?

'Um . . .' floundered Ron, '. . . ah . . . right . . .'

Suddenly they realized the heart monitor was beeping at an almost continuous rate.

Ben turned to Di, horrified.

He hadn't meant . . . He'd been trying to . . .

The door burst open and a nurse rushed in, flung back Ron's sheet, tore down his pyjama pants and jabbed a syringe into his buttock.

Ron slumped back onto the pillow and gradually the beeping slowed back down to a steady rate.

The doctor swept in, checked the reading on the monitor and turned to Di and Ben.

'What on earth did you say to him?' he demanded.

19

FROZEN BEEF?

Di hovered outside the bathroom door wrestling with her conscience.

To listen or not to listen?

Ben had been in there for almost an hour and she was pretty sure he wasn't regrouting the shower cubicle.

Two weeks ago she'd have known what he was doing. Shaving his head and using up another tube of her instant tan lotion. But now she wasn't so sure.

Since the heart attack there had been developments.

The first had been on a wet Saturday afternoon when Ben and Jason were in Ben's room watching a tape and she had taken them in some chips and drinks.

She hadn't even looked at the screen, assuming it would be just another distressing scene of starvation or nuclear suffering. So she'd seen Jason clumsily trying to slide the cassette box out of sight under the bed. And she'd seen the title.

The Last American Virgin.

Then, a couple of days later, Jean had rung

up excitedly to say that she'd just seen Ben walking from the bus stop with young Tracy Anderson from Stringybark Crescent.

Okay, they could just have been talking about homework or instant tan lotion or anything.

Except for the final development.

The extra can of deodorant in the bathroom cabinet.

She had to know what he was doing in there.

What he was doing was standing in front of the bathroom mirror combing the locks of blond hair that curled over his ears and almost fell into his eyes.

It wasn't easy trying to look normal again.

He decided to try the parting on the other side and set to with the comb, tearing it through the stubborn locks with a grimace.

Hair was a real pain after being bald for so long. He didn't know why people bothered. Shampoo, dandruff, split ends. He'd got used to being bald. Still, some people found it harder to cope with. Girls and people.

He stopped combing and looked at the result. He looked like a Wookie. No, nature was going to have to go it alone.

He took off the hair and dropped it in the sink, hoping that Jason would be able to sneak it back into his mother's wig drawer without

Jean noticing they'd trimmed it.

Then he set to with the comb again, trying to get a part in the stubble that covered his scalp.

Outside the bathroom Di's conscience was winning.

She looked at the bathroom door. So easy just to go over and put her ear to it. But she couldn't.

She took one step closer to see if she could hear anything without actually listening at the door. Nothing. Silence.

Then the phone rang and she nearly wet herself.

She snatched up the receiver.

'Hello?'

Probably Jean wanting to yak.

She listened to the few words spoken at the other end and her face filled with delight and amazement. She struggled to keep these emotions out of her voice.

'Er . . . just a moment, please.'

She pounded on the bathroom door. Ben stuck his head out looking startled.

Di looked so casual that if she'd been any more relaxed she'd have nodded off.

'Phone for you,' she murmured. 'Someone called Tracy.'

Ben took the phone and went into his bedroom, closing the door behind him.

Di eagerly pressed her ear to the woodwork.

Two weeks later Ron was able to ruffle Ben's hair for the first time since the fateful barbie.

Ron was sitting up in bed and looking well. There were still bags under his eyes but much smaller than before.

Or as Wal had put it when Ben and Claire bumped into him as he was leaving the ward, 'wallets instead of potato sacks'. They'd left him gathering invoices off the corridor tiles.

'Wish I could grow mine back that easy,' said Ron, when he'd given Ben's hair a ruffle. 'Bet the girls go for it, eh mate?'

Ben looked at the floor and went red.

Some parents just didn't deserve to be kept safe.

'They're just kids from school,' he mumbled.

Claire, whose romantic confidence had increased by bucketfuls since boycotting pizza following the heart attack and actually talking to the boys, stepped in to save Ben.

'We're really looking forward to having you home,' she said to Ron. 'Mum's been getting ready for tomorrow all week. She's got you a great rocker/recliner for the patio.'

Ron flung back his head and roared with laughter.

Ben realized he hadn't seen Dad laugh like that since . . . he couldn't remember. It was going to be great having him at home all day and as he got stronger they could talk and . . .

'The patio?' laughed Ron. 'Tell her if she wants me to recline she'll have to put it in the office.'

Ben felt his heart sink.

20

THE TOPSIDE

It was just as well trail bikes don't get offended easily.

The Welcoming Committee had been lined up on the driveway for hours. The Fairlane, the 'Cutlet Queen' on its trailer, the surf skis and the trail bikes, all gleaming patiently in the sunshine.

Di's Mazda had pulled up and Ron had leapt out and rewarded them with a fond gaze that lasted all of one and a half seconds.

He breathed in a big lungful of air and turned to Di.

'Feels good,' he said.

The trail bikes needn't have worried. There were bricks in his dream home that Ron didn't even look at.

'Sure does,' smiled Di, dropping his hospital bags and giving him a big hug. 'Both my men completely recovered.'

She called up to the house.

'Ben! Ben!'

She turned to Ron, bubbling with delight at having him home.

'He's completely back to normal,' she

gushed. 'It's as if none of that business ever happened.' She gave Ron another hug and dropped her voice in joyful conspiracy.

'I told you about the phone calls from his little girlfriend.' She glanced towards the house to make sure Ben hadn't appeared.

'Well look, look at this, look what I found in his room this morning.'

As she spoke she scampered into the garage and emerged brandishing a bundle of florist's tissue papers wrapped round a few flower stems and stray petals.

'Our son's saying it with flowers,' she beamed.

'Great,' said Ron. 'I'll have a chat with him as soon as I get back.'

Di's face fell.

'Get back from where?'

'The office,' said Ron. He climbed into the Fairlane.

For a second Di thought her ears had taken leave of their senses. Then she realized it was Ron who'd taken leave of his.

'The doctor said absolutely no work for at least three months,' she said furiously. 'And even then, quote "he must on no account re-sume his previous workload".'

Ron revved the Fairlane.

'Easy for him to say,' he said. 'I've got a business to run.'

He blew Di a kiss and drove off.

Di ran down to the Mazda and flung herself

behind the wheel.

Ron strode across the bulkstore, nodding to startled employees he hadn't even met.

He looked around for the signs of sloppiness that sprang up like fungus when a boss was away. Floor scrubbed, all the cold store doors shut, trucks washed, everyone wearing hair covering. Looked pretty good. But then they knew he was coming today.

Di strode alongside him, talking in a low, urgent voice.

'Ron, medical experts have said if you push yourself now you'll die.'

'Negative thinking,' said Ron.

Wal fell into step next to them.

'Er . . . Ron . . .' he said.

Four weeks as a stand-in manager hadn't done anything to stretch his collar and he fingered it nervously as he tried to get Ron's attention.

'For God's sake be sensible,' pleaded Di. 'Doesn't almost being killed by a heart attack mean anything?'

'Almost killed?' Ron was getting annoyed. 'It was a flutter.'

'Er . . . Ron . . .' said Wal. He scrunched the invoice he was holding into a tiny, moist ball.

Ron stopped outside his office door.

'Look, love,' he said to Di, 'I appreciate what

you're trying to do, but I've made up my mind. I'm going to build this company into the biggest meat wholesaler in the state. Those, my love, are the facts of life.'

Di looked at him and her eyes filled with tears.

'Isn't there anything that'll make you see sense?' she begged.

Ron turned away, flung open his office door and stormed in.

The blood drained from his face.

Sitting on his desk was a coffin. Standing next to it, dressed in black, was Claire. Lying in it, his skin stained a deathly blue, was Ben.

Ben sat up, opened his eyes and looked steadily at Ron. He lifted up a home-made gravestone which bore, in ghastly gothic lettering, the words,

'Ron Guthrie. 1944-198? Husband, father, meat.'

Di, who for a moment had looked as if she might keel over from shock, lit up with a delighted smile and went over and stood on the other side of the coffin.

Wal sheepishly shuffled over and stood next to Claire.

Ron stared at them, his mouth open.

Ben, Di, Claire and Wal stared back.

Ron contemplated the battle ahead. He had an awful suspicion who was going to win.

The 'Cutlet Queen' was moored in sparkling blue water under a perfect blue sky.

Di lay on the gently rocking deck feeling the sun soaking into her. She knew she was radiating something out as well.

Happiness.

She glanced over at Ron, who was stretched out between her and Claire. He looked tanned, healthy and content.

She rolled over and nuzzled his ear.

'At last,' she murmured, 'a normal family having a normal holiday.'

Ron didn't open his eyes.

'Hope Wal's remembered to turn up the freezers,' he said.

Di bit his ear.

He opened his eyes.

Di pointed up to the mast.

Lashed to it was the home-made gravestone.

Ron kissed Di on the chin.

'Sorry,' he said.

He reached into her drink, plucked out an ice-cube, dropped it into Claire's navel, waited for her to stop screaming, then called out in the direction of the cabin.

'Come on, Ben, when are you going to tell us our mystery destination?'

Ben bounced up from below decks with an armful of papers and charts. The breeze ruffled his hair.

'Anywhere you like,' said Ron, 'as long as you do the charts and paperwork. Where's it to be? Wollongong? Port Macquarie?'

Ben dropped a bundle of papers onto Ron's chest. There were various important-looking documents with rubber-stamp marks and embossed seals. Plus passports, a wad of banknotes in strange colours and a copy of *Time* magazine.

Ron read the *Time* cover. 'Third World – Helping Them To Help Themselves.'

He looked up at Ben, puzzled.

'Coffs Harbour?'

Ben looked at him steadily.

'Bangladesh.'

While his stunned parents stammered for words to protest with, Ben winched up the anchor, fired up the diesel, took the wheel and, deaf to everything but the ecstatic throb of purpose in his veins, steered the boat out towards the open sea.

YOUR MOTHER WAS A NEANDERTHAL

Jon Scieszka

The dinosaur looked at us and roared again. We went to the Stone Age to become kings, and were about to become lunch.

What better way to avoid doing maths homework than to take a trip (with the help of Joe's magic book) back to the Stone Age. The Time Warp Trio plan to wow their ancestors with modern inventions, like juggling balls, water pistols and Walkmans. But dinosaurs, dangerous cavewomen, tigers, earthquakes and woolly mammoths are just a few of their problems.

'You say there is nothing for boys to read? Can't find anything that mixes adventure, comedy and a tad of hocus-pocus? Never fear, the Time Warp Trio has arrived' – *Booklist*

HANDS OFF OUR SCHOOL!

Joan Lingard

Small is beautiful!

Katy McCree and her friends are in an uproar: their one-teacher school in the Highlands of Scotland might be closed down! Every family in the village becomes involved in the fight to save the school. And by the time spring arrives, the community has come up with a daring plan: parents, pupils and teacher will go to Edinburgh to confront the Director of Education himself — and they even end up on television!

THE FOX OF SKELLAND
Rachel Dixon

Samantha's never liked the old custom of Foxing Day – the fox costume especially gives her the creeps. So when Jason and Rib, children of the new publicans at The Fox and Lady, find the costume and Jason wears it to the fancy-dress disco, she's sure something awful will happen.

Then Sam's old friend Joseph sees the ghost of the Lady and her fox. Has she really come back to exact vengeance on the village? Or has her appearance got something to do with the spate of burglaries in the area?